Dilemmas in Community Mental Health Practice:
Choice or Control

Rachel Perkins

and

Julie Repper

Radcliffe Medical Press

Radcliffe Medical Press Ltd
18 Marcham Road, Abingdon, Oxon OX14 1AA, UK

British Library Cataloguing in Publication Data

A catalogue record for this book is available from the British Library.

ISBN 1 85775 181 7

Library of Congress Cataloging-in-Publication Data is available.

Typeset by Advance Typesetting Ltd, Oxon
Printed and bound by Redwood Books Ltd, Trowbridge, Wilts

Contents

Preface

Mental health services have undergone fundamental changes since the 1960s with the move from an institutional to a largely community-based system of care. Many commentators have described the contradictory role that mental health services have within society (Jones, 1972; Foucault, 1967). Such contradictions are no less evident in community-based services than they were in institutional ones. Different interest groups have always jostled for the right to determine what such services do, and moves to community-based services have simply increased the number of such groups. National and local campaigning bodies, politicians, public agencies like the police and courts, local community groups, purchasing authorities, different provider agencies, managers, clinicians, and the relatives and friends of users all vie with service users to determine what should be provided for them and how it should be provided. The power and demands of these disparate groups vary: keep the community safe, cut the cost of care, make sure people comply with treatment, give service users choice about what happens to them.

Nowhere are such contradictory demands greater than in relation to services for people who are more seriously disabled by their mental health problems. It is not simply service systems which feel the pressure of such contradictions, but individual clinicians of all disciplines in the course of their day-to-day work. Increasingly, clinicians are exhorted to base their practice on scientific evidence garnered in research trials (DoH, 1993c). While this is no doubt important, science and research trials cannot answer many of the ethical dilemmas which face clinicians. Whose views should be prioritized? What should we be trying to do? And why? (Tyrer *et al.*, 1994)

Because of the pressures faced by clinicians, it is not always easy to fully appreciate or explore the value judgements that practice necessarily involves. It is interesting in this context to note that while research can only be conducted with ethical committee approval, there are few clinical ethics committees to guide clinical practice in similar uncharted territory. An absence of consideration of ethical judgements can inadvertently aggravate relationships with other stakeholders in the mental health enterprise, especially those between the central actors: service users and clinicians. It will never be possible to please everyone all the time, but it is important to know why particular decisions are made and what the options might be.

The ethical dilemmas facing clinicians are particularly important in an era when growth of the mental health user/survivor movement has begun to change the balance of power within mental health services. The historically disregarded views and preferences of service users themselves are beginning to take a higher profile. Mental health service users have been involved in hundreds of local action groups and in conferences and training for professionals; the NHS and Community Care Act made consultation with users a necessity; users have given evidence to Department of Health and parliamentary reviews of mental health and have been involved in the Mental Health Task Force and Mental Health Nursing Review (Campbell, 1997). It is our contention that an even larger challenge is now facing mental health services than that involved in the move from hospital to community-based care: whether, at an individual and organizational level, providers can allow those who use services to have choice and control over what they receive and what happens to them. This will involve a fundamental shift in the balance of power which, if not achieved, might result in statutory mental health services becoming increasingly redundant – as users 'vote with their feet' – and increasingly reliant on force to ensure that people use them.

The purpose of this book is to explore a range of dilemmas that typically occur in relation to work with people who are seriously disabled by ongoing mental health problems. Many of these dilemmas revolve around the increasingly vexed issue of 'who should decide': service users themselves, or clinicians, relatives, politicians, the general public...? We do not pretend to have provided an exhaustive account, nor is it possible to write such a text from an entirely neutral perspective. Both of us have been committed for our entire careers to working with people who experience serious mental health problems. Over a combined total of some 30 years our interest and enthusiasm has grown, fuelled by our liking of, and respect for, those whom we serve and a firmly held belief that they have an important contribution to make to our communities. This commitment is not simply driven by professional interest, nor by altruism, but by a belief that people who have serious mental health problems have a right to full citizenship. The communities in which all of us live are poorer places when deprived of the contribution of those who have been marginalized and excluded as a consequence of their mental health problems.

We met each other over a decade ago working in a rehabilitation service in south London: Julie as a nurse, Rachel as a clinical psychologist. Since this time we have worked together and separately in a variety of clinical, teaching and research capacities. After leaving clinical practice to work as a lecturer in nursing studies, Julie became a research fellow in a health services research unit and is now a full-time research student. Rachel began her career as a lecturer and clinician specializing in work with people who experience more serious mental health problems. She is now a consultant clinical psychologist and clinical director of a rehabilitation and continuing care service in London. We have both written widely in the area – including our previous book *Working Alongside People with Long-term Mental Health Problems* (Chapman & Hall, 1996) – presented papers at national and international conferences and provided training for mental health workers from all disciplines and a range of agencies. The ideas we present here come from 15 years of joint and separate work, shared argument and debate, but our understanding of mental health problems does not come from work alone. Rachel herself has a diagnosis of manic depression and was hospitalized for a period during the writing of this text.

This book is written for all those involved in the mental health enterprise. It is primarily intended for practitioners and managers of all disciplines and from all agencies: from trainees and assistants to consultants and senior managers. We hope it will be useful in training – both pre- and post-qualification – in all sectors of the mental health system and that it might be of value to service users, whose views we have explored widely in writing the text. A book such as this is necessarily controversial. We urge the reader not to dismiss the ideas and discussion presented out of hand but to think about them and consider their implications. We hope that this book will inspire thought and debate about what we believe to be some very important areas.

In writing this book we owe a great deal to a large number of people, too numerous to name here. However, we would like to thank Dean Repper for his ideas and comments on the text, our clinician colleagues and the people who have experienced serious mental health problems whom we have had the privilege to know. It is these people who, both in person and through their writing, have acted as our most influential teachers and guides in understanding the ethical dilemmas discussed in this book.

Rachel Perkins
Julie Repper
February 1998

1

Introduction:
a stakeholder economy?
Interests and conflicts

His father is scared of him, after all he has threatened him on many occasions when he has been short of money, but then, he is ill… he should be in hospital where the doctors can help him. His psychiatrist, whilst accepting that he has had a mental illness, is convinced that the robbery he committed had less to do with his mental state than with his desire for drugs… it is for the courts to decide whether he needs a custodial sentence and if so, then prison is the right place for him. If his mental health problems get worse then he can be treated there. The courts see his history of mental illness. They know just how full the prisons are with repeat petty offenders and people with mental health problems, he would be much better off in a mental hospital. This is the last place he wants to be. He knows that there is nothing wrong with him and he will not even consider the idea of voluntary admission. He just wants to be left alone in his own place. The Social Services Department do not agree. He has been evicted from all of their hostel facilities because he has stolen from, and got into fights with, other residents. They are under pressure from the Housing Department because of the enormous rent arrears he has accrued on his current flat. This, combined with the large number of complaints about his behaviour from angry neighbours, has led them to start eviction proceedings… his needs are for 'health', not 'social', care. In desperation, neighbours have written to their MP who has in turn contacted the local Trust providing mental health services and the Health Authority which purchases these services. Not surprisingly they are demanding that 'something' be done.

It is now widely accepted – enshrined in legislation (DoH, 1989b; 1990; 1991a; 1991b) – that mental health services should be based on the 'needs' of service users. While this is undoubtedly a laudable aim, issues immediately arise concerning how these needs should be defined. Need is a relative concept, inextricably bound with notions of 'rights', demands, effectiveness, availability and cost – the example above illustrates the number of groups and individuals who might claim an understanding of a person's 'needs' and the right to speak on their behalf. Although the issues, circumstances and interested parties may vary from one situation to another, in clinical practice it is common for different 'stakeholders' to hold conflicting and competing views about what 'needs' should be provided for, at both individual and service levels.

The list of potential stakeholders is almost endless, from shopkeepers and neighbours, through a plethora of providers of support and services, to the individual who experiences mental health problems. Each group occupies a different position in terms of its role, influence, level of responsibility, accountability and, ultimately, its power, and each encompasses many contradictory beliefs and opinions. Nevertheless, there are some common themes and a distinction might usefully be drawn between potential decision-making groups: the 'patient', the technical expert and society (Williams, 1978). For the purposes of this discussion the first group includes service users, user organizations and user advocates – the people who themselves experience mental distress; the second, providers of formal and informal treatment, care and support; and the third, the general public and public organizations like the police and justice system.

Service users, user advocates and user organizations

Throughout all the discussion, debates and conflicts about mental health services, it is the lives of people with mental health problems that are at stake. It is people with mental health problems who are the subject of the mental health enterprise: they use services and services are set up to address their problems. It might therefore be assumed that these people would be the central stakeholders in determining what is provided for them, and how, when and where it is provided. This is not, however, the case.

McGuire *et al.* (1988) argue that most people, whether they have mental health problems or not, do not have sufficient information to assess *'the relationship between health care and health status'*. Nevertheless, most adults expect to be accorded the right to define their own wants and needs. Although these may not always be met, the right to define them remains. There are likely to be few readers of this book who do not assume the right to receive information and, on the basis of this, make their own decisions about the healthcare they receive. However, when a person has the cognitive and emotional difficulties that characterize mental health problems it is too often assumed that their ability to define their own wants, wishes, problems and needs is diminished. As Torrey (1986), a psychiatrist, demonstrates:

'Assuming… that someone with schizophrenia is capable of making intelligent decisions regarding his or her own needs is like assuming that a person with heart disease has normal cardiac function and can run a marathon.'

Although there are probably few people in the mental health arena who would actually admit to sharing such an extreme perspective, similar attitudes are often implicit. The assumption of diminished ability to make, and take responsibility for, decisions means that if a person has mental health problems then their views, beliefs and ideas are cast into doubt and the prospect of other people speaking for them is raised.

In former times, service users were deprived of the status of stakeholders by simple exclusion. They were absent from all service planning meetings and only invited to ward rounds to demonstrate their symptoms and hear the doctor's prescription. The efforts of an ever-growing user/survivor movement have done much to increase the involvement of service users at both an individual and a service level (Campbell, 1997). Now it is increasingly common for service users and user groups to be involved in service planning, and demands for 'client-centred care' have increased their involvement in care planning meetings and case conferences.

Nevertheless, service users remain a relatively powerless and devalued group and it is still common for them to remain deprived of any real involvement in those very services which centrally affect their lives (Bowl, 1996). The physical presence of users is rarely accompanied by effective collaboration but, instead of exclusion, there exist a variety of ways in which their views of care and services are routinely disregarded (for example Perkins 1996a).

Dismissing the views and ideas of users because they do not agree with each other

'You cannot agree with each other, so we do not know who to believe' (therefore we will do what we believe is best for you). 'You may say that, but many of my [sic] patients agree with me' (so it's all right to carry on as I have been doing). It is very easy to devalue what service users say by pointing out the differences in perspective among them (Crepaz-Keay, 1996). As any collection of individuals, mental health service users are a diverse group representing different cultures, experiences, political beliefs, religions and so forth. They also have a range of different difficulties and experiences of mental health services. This diversity could be viewed as an asset, bringing with it a range of expertise – a rich seam of ideas and knowledge – to mental health services. Instead, it is all too often used as a way of disregarding what users say in favour of other stakeholders: 'If they cannot agree amongst themselves we will have to decide for them'.

Limited resources

'We haven't got the resources' (so we have no option but to carry on as we have been doing). When service users express opinions or ideas it is often assumed that these represent 'the icing on the cake' rather than 'the cake itself'; extras to be pursued only if resources are available. Such an approach clearly places service user stakeholders at the bottom of the heap, only to be heeded in the unlikely event of spare resources being available over and above that necessary to provide the 'core' services – as defined by other stakeholders. The allocation of scarce resources is always a political decision. It would be possible to provide that which users suggest *instead* of that which other stakeholders deem necessary, for example a user-run day drop-in *instead* of an existing day centre. That this rarely happens reflects the relatively powerless status of service users.

Making service users fit in

The 'token user' on an existing committee, with *modus operandae* set by other stakeholders, is inevitably a relatively powerless figure (Conlan, 1996). Even when this individual is accompanied by a group of users, if the terms of reference of the group are set by others, then the user agenda will by definition have to 'fit in' with that of other stakeholders. Unless users themselves set the questions, their opportunities to make their views, wishes and ideas clear are limited by the parameters of issues defined by other, more powerful, groups.

Humouring

'Yes dear, how interesting'. In a climate where the imperative to 'involve' service users is increasingly strong (DoH, 1993a) many other stakeholders spend time 'listening' to users. The real question is whether they *hear* what is said. It is not uncommon for 'listening' to be more akin to humouring – attending politely and taking no notice at all. Alternatively, persuasion may be employed. When a service user expresses a view, it is not uncommon for them to find this refuted in vigorous terms, and the power of verbal persuasion should not be underestimated. In a survey of mental health service users, Lucksted and Coursey (1995) found that 58% reported having been pressured or forced into taking some form of treatment/therapy and that the most common type of force used was verbal persuasion.

You cannot believe what people with mental health problems say

'You only think that because of your delusions/faulty cognitions/disturbed intra-psychic process' (because I am the expert, I know what you really mean better than you do yourself, therefore I will do what I think is best for you). The views, opinions and ideas expressed by service users are often dismissed as an indication of their psychopathology. Most 'professional' models quite arrogantly accord professionals the right to interpret what service users 'really' mean. Within such a framework it stands to reason that the views expressed by service users should be treated with caution and seen as part of their illness. This perspective is not limited to the professional domain. In lay circles the 'does s/he take sugar' approach that has long dogged people with physical disabilities is even more prevalent in relation to those with mental health difficulties. Clearly, if what a person says cannot be trusted then the views of other stakeholders must take precedence.

This professional and popular scepticism results from a belief that, to a greater or lesser extent, such people lack the ability to define their own wants and wishes and need the protection of someone else deciding on their behalf, in their 'best interests'. This effectively denies service users a central role in the mental health arena and other interested parties – professionals, relatives, the general public and so forth – vie for ascendancy in defining what should be provided, where, how and by whom.

Providers of treatment, care and support

As the care and support of people with mental health problems has moved into community settings, increasing numbers of different agencies and professionals are involved in the provision of mental health services. It is often assumed that all these interested parties work in amicable co-operation (Tossell and Webb, 1994) and that a consensus can always be reached. Although it is possible for different agencies and individuals to work together, their different natures, positions and concerns mean that they hold differing views about their roles and what is best for 'their'[sic] clients. If they are to work together effectively, these areas of conflict cannot be swept under the carpet but must be explicitly addressed.

The commissioning role of general practitioners (GPs) makes them increasingly important in determining the nature of secondary mental health services and that which is provided by these services for 'their'[sic] clients. It is assumed that mental health services are the experts in mental health issues while GPs are the experts about the person, their family and circumstances. Both of these assumptions are open to question.

First, it seems to be assumed that everyone is registered with a GP and that GPs have a long and intimate knowledge of all those on their books. There are, however, many people who rarely consult their GP, have no GP or have changed GP regularly, and the consultation times possible in general practice do not always allow full personal and social histories to be taken. Second, mental health services are not monolithic but comprise numerous different professionals with different constructions of mental distress and prescriptions for its relief. Conflicts between these different professionals and agencies, and their prescriptions, are a day-to-day occurrence. Third, because of their different situations, GPs and mental health services tend to focus on different groups of people. Mental health services are obliged to prioritize people with serious ongoing mental health problems (DoH, 1989c; 1991a; 1991b; 1995a), but taken as a whole this group does not make heavy use of GP services. Although those who do use their GP often consult more frequently than do people with other disorders, a substantial proportion either do not have any contact with their GP or avoid contacting their GP even when they have serious difficulties (Meltzer et al., 1991). In terms of time spent, and numbers seen, the mental health work of GPs tends to focus on people who are extremely distressed by less disabling and sometimes more transient anxiety-based problems and depression. Not surprisingly then, it is this group that is often their prime concern when commissioning secondary mental health services. This leaves mental health services facing the often irreconcilable demands of national policy (to prioritize people with serious mental health problems) and GP demands (for quick attention to their distressed but less seriously disabled patients) and leaves GPs feeling ill served by secondary mental health services (Tyrer et al., 1993).

National policy (DoH, 1989a; 1989b; 1989c; 1991a; 1991b) draws a further distinction between 'health' and 'social' care for people who experience serious mental health problems. This is predicated on the assumption that there are some interventions that are clearly treatments for mental health problems (and therefore the responsibility of health services) and some which offer social support to people with ongoing disabilities (and are therefore the responsibility of social services). In reality such a distinction is extremely problematic. People who experience serious mental health problems are particularly sensitive to the social environments in which they find themselves (Brown and Birley, 1968; Falloon et al., 1984; Birchwood et al., 1992). Stressful social circumstances can lead to an exacerbation of their cognitive and emotional problems. Indeed, Warner (1985) demonstrates how low social role, status and social integration of people with a diagnosis of schizophrenia strongly influences the course of their problems. In short, many of the supports which might at first appear to constitute 'social care' – somewhere decent to live, a job, adequate money, good family relationships, acceptance within the local community – are critical 'treatments' for the symptoms of the person's disorder.

The impossibility of drawing clear demarcations between 'health' and 'social' arenas necessarily causes conflicts between health and social care providers. For example, it is not uncommon for social services to deem an individual in need of healthcare because their problems cannot be accommodated by the local authority. However, health services may well argue that there is nothing further that can be done to treat the individual's problems and they require ongoing supported accommodation.

This position is further complicated by differences between statutory authorities and other providers of care and support. Of particular importance in this regard are relatives and friends. Parents in particular, but also spouses and other kin, provide a great deal of ongoing support for people with mental health problems (Kuipers and Bebbington, 1990), but conflicts with statutory agencies are common. While differences may take many forms, they typically revolve around who best knows the needs of the person with mental health problems: the family who are with them day in day out, or the professionals with their expertise in mental health. These differences are often associated with mutual distrust and families feeling that their role is not acknowledged.

As well as statutory organizations and families, voluntary ('not for profit') and private-sector providers also have a major role in the mental health arena. Sometimes these agencies, particularly those in the voluntary sector, have been critical of the 'medical model' and the very notion of 'mental illness' (Davies *et al.*, 1995) on which statutory services base their treatment, care and support. It is not uncommon for conflicts to arise over the appropriateness of different forms of treatment (particularly drugs). Voluntary agencies believe that they can offer care that is less institutional and more sensitive to the needs of the individual than can the statutory sector, but, like families, may feel poorly supported by these statutory bodies in the work that they are doing. On the other hand, it is not uncommon for professionals from statutory agencies to be critical of the way in which the voluntary sector can 'pick and choose' who they take, and often see workers in this sector as being untrained and not really knowing what they are doing. The voluntary sector has also begun to experience some of the public criticism to which statutory services have been subject (Davies *et al.*, 1995) and issues have arisen over the exchange of information between statutory and non-statutory sectors. For example, statutory-sector clinicians have concerns about confidentiality whilst non-statutory-sector workers want full information about people who may have a history of violence.

Conflicts between agencies are exacerbated in a climate of limited resources and imperatives to cut costs and provide value for money. It may be tempting for an agency to argue that some areas of work are the province of another individual or agency in order to decrease pressure on its own budget. Mental health services may try to hand over elements of treatment, care and support to social services or GPs (and vice versa) and it may be in the economic interests of all of these to use the (generally cheaper) voluntary sector or relatives wherever possible. As Muijen and Hadley (1995) describe, the 'buck passing' that is perversely encouraged by such a situation does not make for effective working relationships:

'Why in a system where we may assume all parties have a common interest… is it so easy to find examples of practices which do not seem to service users well? … Quality of care is the

victim of conflicting interests across funding streams. To blame these conflicts on ignorance or even malice is simplistic. The problem is that the incentives built into the current policy structure encourage different priorities for each party. Combined with the shortage of money across agencies, this leads to conflict rather than encouraging co-operation.'

The professionals within any agency have interests of their own which they wish to pursue (*see* Chapter 10): typically they wish to be able to practise their craft – pursue their professional expertise – unfettered by constraints of economics or politics. There are numerous interventions which professionals deem to be effective, many of which are backed by considerable research data. Indeed, there are many who consider research data to be the final arbiter of that which should be provided; if it can be proved effective then it should be offered. In a society which places a high value on science, such arguments wield a great deal of power and are often used to dismiss the demands and views of service users who do not have such a body of research at their fingertips. Unfortunately, there are many problems with this research data. What constitutes effectiveness or proof? How were the studies conducted? And by whom? Were all the possible alternatives evaluated? These are just a few of the questions that might be asked. For example, a particular drug may have been 'proved' to be 'effective' in eliminating a particular symptom, but was this symptom particularly distressing? Are the side effects of the treatment more distressing? Could another intervention have been more effective at decreasing distress, even if it did not get rid of the symptom? That which is of prime concern to clinicians may not be the most important consideration for service users or other interested parties.

As a consequence of the growing user/survivor lobby, political pressure now exists to ensure that treatment, care and support are 'client-centred'; based on the individual's needs and wishes. But these demands are at least matched, and often exceeded, by simultaneous pressures to ensure the protection of the public and the smooth running of communities. Because of the relatively powerful nature of the voices making these latter demands, and the relatively powerless nature of people with mental health problems, the wishes of service users tend to take second place. 'Client-centred' care is rendered an impossibility in the face of conflicting social and political demands. Where service users are given choices, these are usually limited to relatively small details rather than major elements of their care and support.

Communities and public agencies

Some of the most powerful stakeholders in the mental health arena actually exist outside that arena in the form of other agencies (like the courts, police and housing departments) and in the form of individuals and amenities (like shops and pubs) through the power they have to influence politicians and opinion-formers. These public stakeholders are clearly a wide-ranging group with a diverse set of agendas. Nevertheless three themes are evident.

First, there is concern over the protection of the public and the smooth running of communities. The link between madness, dangerousness and disruption is strong in the public mind (Repper *et al.*, 1997). A murder committed by someone who has mental health problems has a more powerful influence on public policy than does one committed by someone without such difficulties or the death by suicide of someone with mental health problems. Indeed, the introduction of the Mental Health (Patients in the Community) Act in 1995, which brought in supervised discharge, constituted one part of a well-publicized government response to widespread public horror following a number of sensationalized homicides by people with mental health problems. This Act was opposed by almost every mental health charity, user, professional and human rights organization in the country. Nursing organizations said the Act was unworkable and The Law Society said it risked contravening the European Convention on Human Rights. Nevertheless, such is the political power of public demand, and such is the political powerlessness of people with mental health problems, that it was introduced anyway.

Alongside the public concern for safety runs a parallel interest in vulnerable people receiving the help and support they need; a belief that 'something should be done' to protect and help the 'poor and needy' who 'cannot help themselves'. The police are often wary of pursuing charges against people with mental health problems and the courts are reluctant to convict them. There is a belief that such people are not really responsible for their wrongdoing; that the courts and prison are not appropriate and that psychiatric hospital care is required instead. Such views are often shared by neighbours and concerned citizens who do not like to see distressed and disturbed individuals within their communities and want to see them helped – for their own good – but preferably in hospital.

The simultaneous support for, and opposition to, community care typifies public responses to 'noxious' facilities (for example sewage works) which are needed and desired but not wanted nearby (Lake, 1983). Such NIMBYism (Not In My Back Yard) has been reported in relation to various marginalized groups: the homeless (Dear and Gleeson, 1991); people with AIDs (Bean *et al.*, 1989); substance abusers and ex-offenders (Fattah, 1982); and people with mental health problems (Repper and Brooker, 1996). A recent survey of public attitudes towards community mental health facilities in England and Wales suggested that local opposition has increased in the past five years, and become more serious in nature (Repper *et al.*, 1997). The main focus of local concern is fear: fear for the safety of children, fear for personal safety, fear of violence and fear that property prices will fall. When the level of misunderstanding and fear among the public is considered alongside the power of the public to influence policy, the need to raise public awareness, respect and acceptance of mental health problems becomes crucial, as does the need to extend legislation ensuring the civil rights of people with mental health problems.

Despite public concern for both their own safety and the well-being of people with mental health problems, mental health services have always received a great deal less funding than physical health services. There are a number of interventions which are known to be effective (the provision of work, Lehman, 1995; intensive outreach work in the community, Stein and Test, 1980, Hoult, 1986; therapy and support for families, Birchwood and Shepherd, 1992; new neuroleptics like Clozapine, Buchanon, 1995), whose availability to those who want them is limited by lack of resources. If similarly effective treatments for physical health problems were known, and not available to those who needed them, there would be a public outcry. Yet public priorities would render it very difficult for a political party to increase the resources available to mental health services at the expense of physical health services. Mental health issues are not popular: the main political concern appears to be the avoidance of potentially embarrassing incidents at minimal expense. And many who might argue for further resources for mental health services (including those who work within services) prefer to keep quiet about their mental health problems or even deny them altogether because of the discrimination that they might face.

A seedbed for clinical dilemmas

There are numerous 'stakeholders' in the mental health arena and somewhere within the rhetoric of each is the claim to be 'acting in the interests of people with mental health problems'. The chapters of this book will explore the ethical dilemmas faced by clinicians working in this situation where numerous 'interested parties' jostle for the right to decide what is done to, and for, those with mental health problems. The various groups and individuals involved often have conflicting interests and each has a different role, influence, level of responsibility, accountability and, ultimately, power in relation to those who are the subject of mental health services: people with mental health problems. The critical question is, therefore, who defines these interests? This issue is problematic because of the way in which people who experience mental health problems, especially serious mental health problems, are understood.

Despite their centrality in mental health services – without them services would not exist – both professional and lay ideas about madness often suggest that it is not really possible to believe what people with mental health problems say. If a person's utterances are merely a manifestation of their problems then their views about their own treatment needs and the nature and provision of services are devalued, and the views of others speaking 'on their behalf' take precedence. These different interest groups and power bases adopt different words and ideas to map the field of mental health. Because of their relatively powerless position, service users often find themselves having to use the language of others in order to make themselves heard: a language that was developed by people who have never experienced the things they are describing.

2

Users, survivors, patients, clients: different words, different meanings

What words should be used to describe those people who experience serious cognitive and emotional problems? How should their problems and the resources provided for them be labelled? Such debates can seem irrelevant to busy clinicians – merely semantics, an affectation of political correctness – but the implications of language should not be dismissed in this way. The language that a person uses gives a clear insight into their attitudes and understanding. Carling (1994) suggests that:

'Historically, language has been the principal tool that has served to separate people with labels of differentness by defining the needs of these people with a label as fundamentally different from those of other citizens. In this way, language keeps oppression intact. Therefore an important way to change these negative stigmatized beliefs and behaviours is to change the language.'

At all levels of service there is an increasing awareness that language matters. The language that we use determines, for example, how services will be viewed by those who need them, how both clinicians and recipients of services view the problems and worth of those who use them, and how efforts to help are understood and valued. In general terms, language is obviously important as it forms the basis of communication between people. But the words used in communication are not merely convenient tags or labels for the things about which we speak. The words that are used, the way in which people and things are named, define roles and power relationships:

'the terms people use to describe their relationship to other people play an important role in creating expectations about the nature of that relationship.' (Mueser *et al.*, 1996)

Alongside a heightened general awareness of the importance of language, specific changes in the mental health arena – particularly the growth of the mental health user/survivor movement – have brought the issue of language to the fore. On the one hand, users are embarking on a process of consciousness raising which involves them coming to a common understanding of what has happened to them and, in effect, creating a language that describes not only their oppression, but their identity. On the other hand, users' concerns about the deleterious and stigmatizing effect of the labels given to people with mental health problems have been rekindled (Chamberlin, 1984). In recognition of the power of language:

'to advance the opportunities for people to come together to find their common voice, and in the short term, to help potential allies change their basic negative assumptions' (Carling, 1994),

the American Psychological Association (1993) has drawn up guidelines for the use of language. These include:

- refer to people as people first and add specific characteristics only as needed
- avoid referring to people as their illness or disability
- avoid extending the nature of their disability (with terms such as 'chronic', 'severely')
- avoid emotionally negative terms (for example 'victim', 'suffering from')
- emphasize abilities, not limitations
- avoid offensive expressions (such as 'psycho', 'crazy')
- avoid metaphoric references to disabilities (for example 'schizophrenic situation')
- refer to people as contributing community members rather than as a burden or a problem.

A further point might usefully be added to this list: avoid 'buzz-words' and jargon. Bachrach (1988b) cites the example of 'community mental health centres' to illustrate the danger of such language. To this phrase might be added 'day centres', 'drop-ins', 'day hospitals' and the shorthand phrases used to describe many services and facilities. Such euphemisms mean different things to different clinicians and almost nothing to uninitiated service users – they are not terms in lay usage – thus they contribute to semantic confusion. There is also a tendency to describe the behaviour and characteristics of individuals using services with jargon, acronyms and reductionist labels: 'delusional beliefs', 'OCD', 'attention-seeking', 'a hoarder', 'a cutter' ... to name but a few. This might provide a convenient shorthand for staff, but it reduces people and their behaviour to preset categories, dehumanizes individuals' experiences and serves to reinforce the barriers between us (the staff) and them (the patients).

There is no simple consensus concerning appropriate terminology in the mental health field (Mueser *et al.*, 1996): indeed in this book we have (mis)used the term 'people with serious mental health problems' as a shorthand for those who are seriously socially disabled as a consequence of their cognitive and emotional difficulties.

Our intention is not to prescribe a 'correct' mental health vocabulary, nor to offer exhaustive consideration of the entire mental health lexicon (this can only be done by those who have experienced the difficulties themselves). Instead, we provide examples of the issues involved by exploring the implications of a range of terms in common usage.

The people and their problems

Numerous different terms have been used to describe people who experience serious ongoing mental health problems and their difficulties: mentally ill, people with mental health problems, people with mental distress and disability, patients, users, survivors, consumers, clients, recipients. A survey in the USA showed that there is no consensus among the individuals to whom these terms refer concerning which is preferable, although the largest proportion (45%) indicated a preference for 'client' (Mueser *et al.*, 1996).

Among the most damaging and criticized terms in the psychiatric lexicon are those which define a person by sole reference to their diagnostic category: schizophrenic, manic depressive and so forth (Chamberlin, 1984). Such language denies the existence of any facet of the person, any relevant roles or characteristics, other than their diagnosis. As Brandon (1991) explains, '... *it is as if the disability dominates the whole person, we can see the wheelchair but somehow the person gets lost'*. A person may have schizophrenia, but they are not 'a schizophrenic'.

This may seem a small distinction but its impact has been far-reaching. Service users and clinicians alike can become unnecessarily hopeless when people are construed solely in terms of their diagnosis: 'I'm just a schizophrenic', 'he or she is just a manic depressive'. If they were to be rid of their problems, what would there be left? It has been suggested that the extent to which a person accepts a diagnostic label affects their prognosis. Scheff (1966, 1975) argued that the public label of mental illness puts pressure on the individual to adopt a self-conception based on a stereotypical image of insanity. Warner *et al.* (1989) found some validity in this argument. In a study of the impact of labels of mental illness, he reported that people who accepted a label of mental illness had lower self-esteem and a reduced sense of self-control. However, in those who accepted their 'illness' label, social functioning was significantly better if they had a sense of personal agency. Evidently people need some understanding of what is happening to them and why, but it is also important for them to know that they are more than just a diagnosis so that they can retain or achieve control over their lives.

In a review of evaluation research into services for people with schizophrenia, Atkisson (1992) attributed recent changes in the nature of service evaluations to this same distinction: when a person is primarily viewed as his or her illness, the success of any service is judged in terms of changes in symptoms as assessed by the psychiatrist. As the social, personal and material needs of people using services are increasingly acknowledged, so service evaluations have increasingly included the views of service users and carers, and the focus of outcome measures has broadened to include social functioning, quality of life, satisfaction with services and so forth.

Although there has been a move away from labelling people solely in terms of their diagnosis, probably the term in most common usage among clinicians remains that of 'patient' with its allied concepts of mental health problems as an illness. The person is not schizophrenic, but they are a patient with schizophrenia. This terminology has the advantage of drawing a clear parallel between mental and physical health problems: it may be argued that if physical illness is not stigmatizing then neither is mental illness. The concept of illness may also carry positive connotations in terms of intervention: illnesses can be treated and cured. However, there are drawbacks.

The role of patient does not carry a high status within our society. Unlike the role of mother or worker it is not positively valued: the person who is a patient is valued only for those roles which they occupy outside the patient role. The patient role is a dependent one: patients are relieved of their everyday responsibilities while they are ill, they do what their doctors say, they rely on other people to make them better. The patient role may be useful when it is temporary and when it comprises only part of an individual's identity. So if someone is ill for a short period, relief from responsibilities is a positive thing, after which a person can return to their usual roles (worker, mother, friend …). If a person has longer-lasting problems, the role of patient may still be useful if they simultaneously occupy other roles. So if someone has an ongoing illness, such as diabetes, they may be a long-term patient in relation to this but simultaneously occupy other valued roles – father, businessman, footballer.

The major problems arise when the role of patient becomes permanent and takes the place of all other roles. This is typically what happens when someone has serious ongoing mental health problems: the interventions used do not fully remove the problems and the person gradually loses the family, work and social roles they previously occupied. Sometimes these roles are lost completely, at other times they are distorted to a point where they are barely recognizable so that the person has no role other than that of 'patient' within their family and social relationships. When the role of patient becomes all-pervasive in this way, the lack of personal agency, lack of self-determination and lack of inherent value in the role become destructive. The person is seen as relatively helpless and dependent by others and often by themselves as well.

Attempts to draw a parallel between mental and physical illness are beset by three types of problem. First, the way in which society constructs illnesses of the body and illnesses of the brain is quite different. A person with illnesses of the body is more often assumed capable, because of their intact capacity for thought, of either making or contributing to decisions about what should happen to them. This is not the case when someone is considered to have an illness of the brain and therefore an impaired capacity for thought and decision-making. This imbalance can be seen in the existence within the Mental Health Act of provision for compulsory treatment for which there is no parallel in physical medicine.

Second, the concept of 'illness' carries with it the assumption of a clear underlying physical pathology. While some people would argue that this is the case with mental illness, others take exception to such notions preferring to stress the social and psychological contributors to mental distress and disability. Although the term 'mental health problems' increasingly replaces that of 'mental illness', the two are barely distinct. There can be no concept of health without one of ill health or illness and what is a health problem if not an illness?

Third, it could be argued that serious mental health problems are more akin to physical disability than physical illness. When a person has a physical illness that cannot be fully remedied they are deemed 'disabled'. They cease to be 'ill' or a 'patient' but instead take on the role of a disabled individual who must build their life within the constraints that their physical limitations (mobility or sensory problems) and the social world (poor access arrangements, being treated as barely human by others) dictate. There are no cures as such for serious mental health problems. There may be a variety of pharmacological, psychological and social ways in which a person's cognitive and emotional problems may be reduced, but they are in the same position as someone with physical disabilities. They must rebuild a life within the constraints of the social disabilities resulting from their mental health problems, e.g. concentration problems, fluctuating mental state, difficulties in thinking and unusual ideas and experiences, and the social disadvantage, prejudice and exclusion that are typically a consequence of the experience of mental health problems in our society (Wing and Morris, 1981; Shepherd, 1984; Perkins and Repper, 1996).

The language of disability – mental distress and disability, psychiatric disability – is useful because it removes the dependency of patient status and introduces the concept of agency (they may receive help, but at the bottom line a person has to rebuild their own life). It also extends horizons by focusing on issues of access. Unlike the 'cures' necessitated by 'illnesses', which essentially involve changing the individual, the 'access' necessitated by 'disability' centrally involves changing the environment in which the person functions to accommodate them.

A further problem of labelling people in terms of their experiences – be they called mental illness, mental health problems or disability – is the implication that there is some group which shares important characteristics in addition to the fact that they have been labelled. As Blanch (1991) points out, given the lack of consensus about the definition and causes of 'mental illness' and given the variable reliability of diagnosis, it may be reasonable to conclude that the only common characteristic of this group is that they have been labelled as 'mentally ill'.

Another set of descriptors come not from the problems which a person experiences, but from their relationship or contact with services. Here there are terms such as 'service users', 'survivors', 'consumers', 'clients' and 'recipients'. Although there are many similarities between these labels, there are also important differences. For example, the terms 'users', 'consumers' and 'clients' imply a voluntary receipt of services. The person chose to use or consume services, or consult as a client. While this may be true for some of the people receiving services, it is not the case for all. Compulsion and involuntary treatment does exist and it is hard to describe someone who is compulsorily detained as a consumer or user of services in the same way as one who uses a supermarket.

Similarly, the terms 'consumer' or 'client' have grown out of attempts to increase the market in mental health provision. Both terms imply that a person has a choice. A consumer can go from one shop to another until they get the things they want. A client of a solicitor or financial advisor can similarly withdraw their custom and go elsewhere if they are not happy with what is offered. To call someone who uses statutory mental health services a consumer or a client is probably inaccurate as few have any meaningful choice over what they receive: without the funds for private help there is nowhere else to go if they don't like what is on offer in their local service.

The terms 'user' and 'survivor' have connotations that reflect their different origins. Both came from the movement of people who had themselves experienced mental health difficulties. The term 'user' is one often adopted by a more 'reformist' wing of this movement whose aim is to improve the quality of mainstream services offered. The term 'survivor' is one adopted by people who see themselves as having survived the mental health system and all the negative experiences associated with it. It is a term that conveys a more activist, campaigning stance and is often adopted by the more radical wing of the user/survivor movement whose aim is not only to create radically different alternatives to existing provision, but also to change the status of users/survivors within society as a whole through public education, influencing the media and developing their own understanding of devalued areas of personal experience (Campbell, 1997). Others prefer the term 'recipient'. This is intended to identify one who receives mental health services without indicating that they have any choice in the matter; the mere receipt of input whether voluntary or compulsory.

Despite these differences, words that describe people who experience serious mental health problems in terms of their relationship to services – whether they be client, survivor, user, consumer or recipient – share a common difficulty. They cannot be used to describe those people who, despite their mental health problems, have not used or actively avoid mental health services: a group who have been the cause of much concern (Hirsch *et al.*, 1992). This means that this latter group are simply not named. As Mary Daly (1978) has argued, the power of naming is not only to define the quality and value of that which is named, it is also to deny the reality of that which is not named. If those who avoid current services are not named, then there is the risk that they will not be considered in rendering services more appropriate to the needs of those who require them.

Cures and the therapy culture

The process of change generally allied to the popular illness constructions of mental health difficulties is one of 'cure': the treatment of assumed underlying causes that arrests the development of, or eliminates, the symptoms that characterize the illness. Most mental health professionals receive a training that is broadly cure-based (Perkins and Dilks, 1992; Ekdawi and Conning, 1994; Perkins and Repper, 1996). Within a variety of models – organic, cognitive, psychotherapeutic, analytic, systemic and so forth – underlying problems or symptoms are identified. Steps are then taken to put things right – reduce or get rid of the symptoms – using a variety of therapeutic interventions like medication, psychotherapy, counselling and family therapy.

This type of cure-based language has the major advantage that it can engender optimism and hope. The belief that all problems can be eliminated offers a positive view for both service user and clinician who may then be motivated to work for change – that is, until it becomes evident that none of the 'cures' available are likely to eliminate the difficulties that the person faces. In the face of such ongoing disability, cure-based approaches can readily become a council for despair which Deegan (1992) describes as a:

'winter of anguish that… is hell not only for those living in it, but also for the ones who love and care for us: friends, families and even professionals.'

If the change process is understood solely within the language of cures, this implies that the only way a person can lead a meaningful and happy life is by getting rid of their problems. Such a perspective has several negative effects. First, it implies that life with a disability is not worth living. That someone who has lost the use of their legs, or has thinking and concentration difficulties, is somehow a 'lesser being' whose life can never be worthwhile. Second, it implies that the only change possible is within the individuals themselves (or in their family/network in the case of systemic models). This means that it completely ignores the social disadvantages and environmental influences that limit a person's life possibilities and exacerbate their disabilities (Wing and Morris, 1981; Perkins and Repper, 1996; Davey, 1994). Third, it precludes the possibility that aspects of what have been described as mental health 'problems' are valuable and meaningful for the individual concerned. There are unknown numbers of people who would not wish to get rid of their mental health 'problems' even if they could (Jamison, 1995). Fourth, the status attached to cure-based models has led to a prioritization of treatment over support, care and environmental manipulations.

Normalization theorists (Wolfensberger and Tulman, 1982) have described how this primacy accorded to treatment and cure has ensured that every activity of life within mental health services has become some form of therapy or acquired a spuriously technical label. First, everyday activities such as talking, bathing, washing and cleaning one's room have become counselling, self-care and home management. This is not simply a semantic shift: counselling and home management imply higher status activities than talking, hoovering and dusting. However, this change of label has the effect of setting the 'mental patient' apart from other people: how many of those outside mental health services do home management and self-care? How many are being counselled when they talk about their activities, aspirations and fears to their friends and loved ones?

Second, all manner of daily activities have become transformed into therapies: work becomes work therapy, a variety of activities and hobbies become occupational therapy, gardening therapy. Once again, the change of name changes the nature of the activity. For example, when an activity is called work this implies that the worker is doing something, or producing something, that is of use or value to someone else. When this activity becomes work therapy, there is no such implication. The primary purpose of therapy is to benefit the person who is receiving it, so the primary purpose of work therapy is to benefit the worker not those who use their products or services. This transformation therefore immediately devalues that which the worker is doing.

A final problem with the primacy of 'therapy' and 'cure' as the means of change is that therapy is typically a time-limited enterprise. Certain interventions are attempted in order to remove a person's problems. If, after a decent trial, the difficulties are not removed, then the therapy is stopped and deemed a failure. It is entirely possible for that which is called therapy to be effective in enabling a person to do things (like work) whilst they are receiving it, but when it is removed they are unable to continue on their own (i.e. gain a job outside a mental health setting unsupported). In the face of ongoing disability, a different construction is required which allows the concept of ongoing interventions aimed at enabling a person to do things that they would not otherwise be able to do: a concept of support and prosthetic aid rather than treatment and cure. A wheelchair or a ramp are not 'therapy' for someone who is physically disabled – neither is help to shop and cook or engage in activities for someone who is socially disabled.

In developing their own language and ideas, users and survivors have adopted the concept of 'recovery' in place of 'cure' and 'treatment': a continuing process of growth and adaptation to disability as opposed to time-limited interventions directed at symptom removal:

'Recovery does not refer to an end product or a result. It does not mean that one is 'cured'. In fact recovery is marked by an ever-deepening acceptance of our limitations. But now, rather than being an occasion for despair, we find our personal limitations are the ground from which spring our own unique possibilities. This is the paradox of recovery, i.e. that in accepting what we cannot do or be, we begin to discover who we can be and what we can do. Thus, recovery is a process. It is a way of life. It is an attitude and a way of approaching the day's challenges.'
(Deegan, 1992)

Recovery involves not only the process of recovering from mental health problems, but also from the effects of discrimination, second class citizenship and the 'spirit-breaking' effect that the use of the mental health system can have (Deegan, 1988; 1990; 1992).

Deegan (1992) describes how:

'We are pressing back against the tide of hopelessness. We are learning that those of us with psychiatric disabilities can become experts in our own self-care, can regain control over our lives, and can be responsible for our own individual journey of recovery... we are learning that the environment around people must change if we are to be expected to grow.'

Similarly, Pembroke (1997) writes:

'I am a person who hears voices and sees visions... I am no longer a victim of any illness or disorder because I decided I wanted a life, and that my voices and self-harm are part of that life however much psychiatrists wanted to deny their existence or remove them... This means accepting the need to self-harm as a valid means of survival, until survival is possible by other means.'

And Harp (1991) explains:

'I have a condition that is neither positive or negative – it cannot be cured. However I can accommodate it in order to enable me to live the way I choose.'

Power or empowerment?

Issues relating to power have been a matter of concern within mental health services for some considerable time, and in particular the lack of power that users of services have *vis-à-vis* the providers of those services (Chamberlin, 1977; Chamberlin, 1990; Campbell, 1996a; Bowl, 1996; Read and Reynolds, 1996). However, this is another area where the language used may be important.

Throughout the literature the terms 'power' and 'empowerment' appear to be used as if the two were interchangeable. Leader (1995), for example, entitles his collection of self-assessment tools (to enable users to work out what they want from services) *Direct Power.* Barker and Peck (1996), on the other hand, in their article on a decade of users working to obtain a voice in British Mental Health Services, adopt *User Empowerment* ... in their title. It is probably true to say that the term 'empowerment' is now more popular in a mental health context than is power. However, it is also the case that power and empowerment have different meanings.

Power is a political term and refers to structural conditions and power relationships between groups and individuals. Power cannot be changed without changes in these structural conditions: change in the rights accorded to different groups. It is these power relationships which Campbell (1996a) describes in his paper *Challenging Loss of Power*:

'I object to the way in which power is stripped from me… The psychiatric system is founded on inequality. By and large, the user is at the bottom of the pile. Our unequal position is symbolised by the compulsory element in psychiatric care. I do not intend to argue either for or against the use of legal compulsion in treatment. But the fact of its existence has repercussions for all service users… That an individual can be compelled to receive psychiatric treatment affects each inpatient regardless of whether their stay is formal or informal… the threat of legal compulsion may be used to coerce individuals to accept particular treatments.'

Unlike the political concept of power, the term empowerment is a psychological one. In empowerment, power is represented not as a set of structural relationships, but as an internal, individual possession (Perkins, 1996a; Kitzinger and Perkins, 1993; Kramarae and Teichler, 1985). Empowerment means the feeling of being powerful, and realizing the power that one already has, rather than changing structural conditions in order to gain more power. Therefore, in the move from power to empowerment, power is redefined as a state of mind in which service users feel more powerful, competent and able to influence events, while leaving the structural inequalities and power relationships, of which Campbell (1996a) speaks, unchanged.

This shift from a political to an individual – psychological – concept can lead to the illusion of power and choice in situations where users actually have no choice at all. It is relatively common for users to be asked what they want and then told that their wishes are 'unrealistic'. One commonly used needs assessment instrument, the *Camberwell Assessment of Need* (Phelan *et al.*, 1995), separately rates the clinician's and user's view of the latter's need in each area, so the user can say what they think they need. However, the assessment gives no indication about how the user's views should be weighted *vis-à-vis* those of the clinician. In the face of the structural inequalities that exist, there is nothing to stop the clinician ignoring what the person says unless, of course, they agree with them.

The whole exercise, like so many others in mental health services, provides a feeling of power – user empowerment – that can never be a reality while structural inequalities remain. To be told that one has a say, has power, when in fact one does not, can be more damaging than simply to be denied power. The blame for *not* getting what one wants rests with the person, e.g. 'We gave you a choice, but you were unrealistic' (some fault in you), rather than with the power structures that maintain the system, e.g. 'You have to do this as you are compulsorily detained' (some fault of 'the system'). Helping people to feel more powerful – empowerment – should not be confused with real structural changes that alter the balance of power. One approach which attempts to help people examine the impact of personal, social and political structures and events on their lives – thus reducing self-blame – is 'power-mapping'

(Hagan and Smail, 1996). Although this technique has not been widely used and evaluated, it has effectively enabled individuals and groups to identify the personal and social changes that are necessary for them to live the lives they wish to lead.

Language and devalued citizens

Although the words used to describe people with mental health problems and the services they receive are important, the power of naming cannot change the world. There is an interaction between the value attached to the person or thing and the language that is used to name it. There have been numerous attempts to change the value attached to people and things by changing the names that are used, e.g. The Spastics Society being renamed SCOPE, mental retardation being renamed learning difficulties and so forth. While such changes can be positive, there is also a tendency for the new label to become devalued because of its association with a devalued group. For example, in the field of mental health, the term 'asylum' was first used to convey the positive image of safety and freedom from the stresses and strains of everyday life. But it was not long before it became associated with institutions and the negative practices they harboured. In mental health parlance, the term 'asylum' now has negative connotations while at the same time in other contexts – oppressed, persecuted and endangered people fleeing from one country to another – it retains its positive associations. The name 'asylum' and the context interact to confer meaning and value.

Similarly, there have been moves towards more positive connotations by changes in terminology from 'mental illness' to 'mental health'. Just as in other areas where, for example, the Department of Employment primarily deals with *un*employment, it remains the case that the Department of Health and Mental Health Services, primarily deal with *ill* health and mental *ill*ness. Indeed, there are many who now use the term 'mental health' as if it were 'mental illness'. As one service user (cited in Repper *et al.*, 1997) said:

'Well my mental health started when I was 15... it stopped me doing things.'

She was not talking about how well she was!

Another strategy in relation to language that has been adopted by several oppressed and devalued groups has been to celebrate and campaign to change, the meaning attached to a devalued label. Among those users/survivors involved in campaigning in the mental health field it is now possible to see a reclaiming of the term 'mad' in this way.

Changes in attitudes towards people with mental health problems will undoubtedly take a great deal more than semantic sleights of hand. Combating the discrimination, degradation and devaluation experienced both within and outside services involves more than a changing of names. However, a recognition of the role of language used and the meaning and values it implies is important at every level from working with individuals to designing and running services. Words carry implications for the way in which people, problems and interventions are construed that cannot be ignored.

3

Who should be served?
The deserving and the
undeserving

The situation in which everyone who experiences mental distress or disability receives all the support that they want or need is neither likely nor feasible. Typically, services have a limited pool of resource and must employ relative judgements about who should receive support and how much they should receive. Usually, the issue is not whether a person needs help or assistance, but whether they are more deserving of support than someone else. To arrive at such decisions, services adopt criteria to determine the priority accorded to different types of difficulties. However, any consideration of who is most appropriately served by mental health services raises fundamental questions about the nature of mental health and the role of services. The manner in which these questions are addressed is important at both a macro, societal, level in determining public policy and at a micro level in the design of individual services and decisions about whether or not a particular person should be offered help and support.

First, there are questions about how to define 'madness': whether a person's thoughts, feelings and behaviour constitute a problem or are simply an acceptable part of human experience. Second, issues arise concerning whether the problem is one of 'madness' or 'badness' – and thus whether it should properly be seen as the preserve of health or criminal and penal services. Third, owing to the division of responsibility for health and social care, questions must be asked about whether the difficulty is of a 'health' or 'social' nature. Finally, for those considered to have 'health' problems, decisions must be made about which service is most appropriate. Demarcation disputes frequently arise in relation to such problems as pre-senile dementia, degenerative disorders such as Huntington's chorea, Korsakoff's psychosis and other alcohol-related brain damage. Problems can also occur concerning the service best suited to an older person with mental health problems or someone who has learning disabilities and mental health problems.

Madness or 'ordinary human distress'?

Mental health services are designed to ameliorate mental distress and disability. However, questions will always arise about how extreme or unusual distress must be – how different from ordinary human misery – to justify intervention. Similar issues arise in assessing when behaviour is sufficiently outside the ordinary range in a particular society – sufficiently different from simple eccentricity and acceptable diversity – to warrant intervention.

The definition of 'mental health problems' is essentially a social one. While some forms of 'madness', akin to diagnoses of major mental health problems like schizophrenia, can be found in most societies (Warner, 1985), others are less widely recognized. Differing definitions of 'normal' behaviour and experience, and differing resources, lead to different definitions of madness and diagnostic practice (Fernando, 1991). Thus there are different cultural, international and political attitudes regarding the diagnosis and treatment of 'problems' such as post-traumatic stress disorder, premenstrual syndrome, homosexuality and a variety of stress-related difficulties.

In the present political climate two contradictory trends can be discerned. On the one hand there has been a wholesale translation of political problems and everyday miseries into psychological problems in need of therapeutic solutions. So, for example, in the USA a group of 22 professionals spent three years and the equivalent of nearly half a million pounds showing how lack of self-esteem is the root cause of *'many of the major social ills that plague us today'* (Reed, 1990). Gloria Steinem (1992) argues that low self-esteem afflicted Hitler, Saddam Hussein, Ronald Reagan, George Bush and entire nations like Haiti and Argentina. Disaster psychologists have been hired in response to environmental disasters like the Exxon Valdez oil spill because of their *'expertise in attending to the special needs of communities struck by tragedy'* (Walker, 1989). And racism becomes a thing to get off one's chest in counselling (Green, 1987).

As Kitzinger and Perkins (1993) argue, it is not only the major political and social issues which are now considered in psychological terms. At an individual level concepts like 'self-esteem', 'inner child' and 'toxic parents' are used:

'We have learned to frame our problems in psychological terms, and to expect psychological solutions to them... turned to psychology because this is one of the dominant culturally available frameworks for thinking about experience.'

Because problems have been increasingly construed in psychological terms – as mental health problems – there has been an increased demand for mental health solutions in the form of therapy and counselling.

On the other hand, in an economic climate of limited public resources, an opposite trend can be discerned. There appears to be a raising of the threshold for defining problems in need of intervention (DoH, 1995a). Those with more 'serious and enduring' problems are deemed to have priority in relation to statutory services at the expense of those whose distress may be just as severe but considered more transient or less disabling in nature. This can mean that distress that is labelled 'neurotic' rather than 'psychotic' goes unaddressed. Barnes (1996) has argued that this may differentially disadvantage women as they are more likely to have 'neurotic' diagnoses (anxiety, depression) and in particular those who have been sexually abused (Briere and Runtz, 1987). As Barnes (1996) argues:

'When distress is described as "neurotic" it can be made to appear trivial. The term "neurotic" can be used as a term of abuse by mental health workers, as well as others, and when it is combined with the term "housewife" the stereotype is complete.'

Around 23% of the population go to their GP with some form of diagnosable mental health problem at some time in their lives (DoH, 1993b). If this figure is added to the undoubtedly substantial number who experience mental distress but do not consult their GP, the potential pool of people with mental health problems who may be deemed to need help is very large. That the demand for help for the increased number of difficulties deemed to be mental health problems is not fully addressed within statutory services can be seen in the ever-growing number of counsellors and therapists in the private sector and the increasing range of therapies they practise. As such therapy must be paid for, and even the most 'sliding' of fee scales are beyond the reach of the poorest in society, this means that access to help for that distress which is considered less serious is available only to the more affluent. Although there have been calls for therapy to be more 'accessible' to disadvantaged groups, this over-simplifies the issue.

When ordinary human misery is defined as a mental health problem in need of specialist help, it is necessarily individualized and pathologized. Distress in response to the vicissitudes of life comes to be seen not as an ordinary part of the human condition but as undesirable and unnecessary – something to be cured (Kitzinger and Perkins, 1993). At a more ludicrous extreme it has been suggested that perhaps everyone should take the anti-depressant Prozac because it would make them feel better than well! Or, as Orbach (1996) 'jokes':

'If you are anxious you need to see an analyst. If you aren't anxious, you definitely need to see an analyst.'

Social problems such as unemployment, discrimination and social isolation become individual difficulties requiring not social but individual solutions in the form of therapy. Distress is increasingly seen as the specialist preserve of experts – therapists, psychiatrists, counsellors. Communities and families no longer expect to support their neighbours and relatives in times of distress, and increasing amounts of ordinary misery are consigned to the private realm of the doctor, counsellor and therapist. The social costs of the pathologization of increasing amounts of ordinary misery, as well as the simple monetary ones, are important.

Madness or badness?

When a person's behaviour strays outside that which is deemed 'acceptable' by the society in which they live, questions arise concerning whether they acted as they did because they were in some way 'mad', and therefore in need of treatment, or because they were 'bad', and in need of punishment (or some form of religious exorcism). Although matters are rarely as clear cut as this (much behaviour being seen as a product of differing combinations of the two) it would appear that there is a tendency to favour 'madness' explanations and 'treatment' disposals over 'badness' explanations and 'punishment'.

In an era when prison populations are rising alarmingly, there is an increasing desire to ensure that no-one is inappropriately placed there. It is often deemed inappropriate for those with mental health problems to go to prison, even if those mental health difficulties had little bearing on the crime for which they were charged. If the person is deemed to be dangerous and in need of containment, then a secure hospital facility, not a prison, may be employed. Thus behaviour that would formerly have been considered criminal and punished is now typically seen as a consequence of mental health problems and treated. Anger and violence may once have been seen as bad behaviours over which a person should exercise self-control. Now a more common response is to explore the underlying reasons for such actions in the person's psyche, possibly in a therapeutic setting. For example, sexual violence against women may be addressed by establishing 'social skills training', 'anger management' and 'men's violence' groups. Such 'treatments' are available to rapists in many prisons in England and Wales (in 60 jails according to Carvel, 1991).

Some of those diverted from the crimino-legal system to the health system are people whose crimes are not severe. They are people who undoubtedly have difficulties, need help and who may not be able to cope with the rigours of a prison regime (although interestingly the rigours of a psychiatric hospital regime, especially that in a secure hospital facility, are rarely considered). Often such people face numerous social difficulties and have few personal, social or material resources: poor education, poor housing, homelessness, disrupted family relationships, a history of abuse, extremely limited social networks, poverty and unemployment are common. However, at the present time, social explanations of deviant behaviour are rarely invoked, implying as they do a need for major social change. Explanations in terms of individual pathology are favoured: 'the world as a whole is all right; this one, mad, rotten apple was the problem; after all most homeless people, unemployed people... do not do things like that'.

It also seems to be the case that disturbing and heinous acts of violence – like vicious and apparently senseless sexual abuse and murder – are rarely explained in terms of the perpetrator's badness. Instead, popular perception tends to prefer the explanation that the person was 'mad': preferably mad before the crime, if not, at least odd and different in retrospect but certainly mad at the time (Philo *et al.*, 1994a). This has the advantage of clearly dividing and rendering distinctly different the perpetrator of the dreadful deed from all other people – after all, anyone can be bad, but only 'mad people' can be mad. Empirical research (Cumming and Cumming, 1957) and analysis of media reports (Fattah, 1982) are testimony to the public's general belief that 'the mentally ill' are not on the same continuum as the 'mentally healthy' but are a distinctly different category of being. This type of logic both renders the world a safer place to live (only mad people do dreadful things) and obviates the need for lengthy consideration of why and how a society could produce people who do awful things. The solution becomes simple, lock up mad people because they are dangerous – the increased demands for which can be seen in numerous popular fora (Philo *et al.*, 1994b; Zito Trust, 1995) – usually combined with assertions that community care has 'failed'.

It may be desirable that inappropriate incarceration in prisons be avoided, but perceptions of the relative merits of forcible detention in prison and psychiatric hospital vary. While professionals seem to consider hospital to be a preferred option, it is worth noting that many service users are of the opinion that they would rather go to prison than be compulsorily detained in hospital. As one patient detained in a UK special hospital said:

'... I am a medical hostage. Send me to prison and let me do my time.' (Owen, 1997)

It is clearly desirable that those people who commit offences receive treatment for any mental health problem they have, just as they should receive treatment for physical health problems. The balance between criminal responsibility and mental health problems may be a fine one, but the confounding of mental health problems and legal detention for a crime can be problematic.

The tendency for criminal behaviour to be defined as 'mad' increases the popular association between madness and dangerousness. This association has fuelled public opposition to many community care initiatives and rendered communities increasingly hostile to those in their midst who have mental health problems (Repper *et al.*, 1997), especially those with more serious difficulties (Johannsen, 1969; Bord, 1971). The more that ordinary psychiatric hospitals are used for compulsory detention, the more they take on the role of jails and are seen as places within which everyone has some criminal association. In short, the psychiatric hospital takes on the role of a prison designed to keep the public safe. This is likely to lead to increased reluctance to enter hospital voluntarily and thus to increased compulsion, as well as increased role confusion for professionals. The roles and responsibilities of mental health professional/nurse and jailer are quite different and generally incompatible (Perkins and Repper, 1996).

A greater separation of legal detention for a crime and help with mental health problems could result in those with serious mental health problems who are imprisoned failing to receive the help they need – but this does not have to be the case. If someone who experiences mental health problems commits a crime (or if someone who commits a crime develops mental health problems) then two decisions are necessary: one relating to detention, another relating to treatment/support. Issues of detention are a matter for the courts and custody might properly remain with the penal system. Issues of treatment and support for mental health problems are clinical issues and might properly remain with the mental health system. As with other facets of community care, such help could be provided in the 'community' where the person resides: in the prison community if this is where they are. Government policy to provide local services (DoH, 1989b; 1989c; 1995a) might include the localities within prisons. As in other localities, the range of necessary provision might include acute admission facilities, longer-term residential units, outpatient and day patient services.

While issues of national policy clearly influence the options available to individual teams, it is not uncommon for clinicians to discuss whether a particular individual's disruptive behaviour is 'mad' or 'bad' (Repper and Perkins, 1994; Perkins and Repper, 1996; Breeze and Repper, 1998). Implicit in such discussions is a concern about whether a person's undesirable behaviour was under their control – whether they 'did it deliberately' – or whether they did it because of their mental health problems and 'could not help it'. Generally, the implication is that if they 'could not help it' then they need treatment and understanding. If they 'did it deliberately' then they are unworthy of help and need at best to be admonished for what they have done, and at worst denied or excluded from the service.

Unfortunately, such considerations rarely take into account the interplay of influences on behaviour – social, psychological, psychiatric, situational – and the fact that a simple bipolar distinction between 'madness' and 'badness' can probably never be drawn. No-one operates purely on the basis of 'free will' and everyone's choices are to a greater or lesser extent constrained by internal and external events. Similarly, everyone, no matter how serious their mental health problems, exercises some choices over what they do. To reduce such complexity to a 'mad or bad' judgement is rarely useful although it does provide a basis for excluding a troublesome individual from services: one way of rationing who does and who does not deserve access to limited resources. Often it simply ensures that the person can go and be 'troublesome' elsewhere in their search for help: social services, housing services, voluntary services, family and neighbours.

A problem, but whose problem?

While an individual may be construed as clearly having a problem, even a mental health problem, there are questions to be asked about the nature and, to some extent, the origins of that problem. In particular, many psychiatric and psychological difficulties may be construed as social in nature. For example, there is a wealth of evidence to suggest that eating disorders are significantly affected by social pressures on women to be thin (Orbach, 1992) and that much depression and anxiety is a consequence of unemployment (Smith, 1985) or lack of social support, poor housing and social conditions (Brown and Harris, 1978). Clearly, if a person's difficulties arise from their unemployment or poor housing then a job or a decent place to live would be more appropriate interventions than individual treatment and therapy.

However, it is often argued that despite equal pressures to be thin, all women do not develop anorexia and not everyone who is unemployed or lives in a high rise flat becomes depressed. Therefore it must be something about the individuals who succumb that is important, rather than their social situation. If so it is appropriate to treat these individuals to enable them to cope with their social circumstances. In this context it is useful to consider a parallel situation in physical medicine. If, instead of unemployment, auto-immune deficiency syndrome (AIDS) were considered, there would be little doubt that the HIV virus causes AIDS. The fact that everyone who comes into contact with the virus does not become HIV-positive, that those who do test positive do not all go on to develop full-blown AIDS, and that people with other diseases of the immune system suffer similar effects to those who are HIV-positive does not change the causal role of the HIV virus and AIDS.

Just as with physical health problems, there is undoubtedly an interplay between individual characteristics and resources and the extent to which a person develops mental health problems when faced with adverse circumstances. The impact of life events and social stressors are as evident in relation to the cognitive and emotional difficulties that have been called serious mental health problems (e.g. schizophrenia and manic-depressive disorder), as they are in relation to depressive and anxiety-based difficulties (Birchwood et al., 1992). While it may be important to ensure that an individual has the personal, social and material resources they need to best cope with the effects of life stressors like unemployment, it would be folly to ignore the role of removing the stressor itself – unemployment – in remediating the problem.

In an attempt to formally recognize the role of health and social factors in relation to mental health, the British community care legislation (DoH 1989c; 1991b) has drawn an explicit distinction between health components of care (the responsibility of health services) and social components of care (the responsibility of social services). This represents a positive attempt to ensure that the range of an individual's needs are met by allocating different agencies different responsibilities. However, this distinction is also predicated on the rather naive assumption that it is actually possible to delineate precisely that which is 'health' and that which is 'social' care.

On the one hand social factors apparently do have a direct impact on mental health. For example, it is known that unemployment can cause depression and suicide – an explicit 'mental health' target in government policy (DoH, 1993b) – and the incidence of depression and suicide is higher among those who are unemployed (Platt and Kreitman, 1984). Conversely, mental health interventions can have a direct impact on social functioning, as in therapy to alleviate agoraphobia or decrease the impact of psychotic symptoms. Thus it is often very difficult to distinguish 'health' and 'social' care. Is the provision of work opportunities health care (decreasing suicide and depression) or social care? Is the provision of neuroleptics health care or social care (increasing ability to function in social roles, decreasing need for specialist housing, day and outreach support)?

Relationships between physical and mental health services can be no less problematic. First, there are questions about who should be responsible for the care and support of people with Korsakoff's psychosis, Huntington's chorea, early dementia and so forth. Such problems are particularly acute when the rare occurrence of a condition precludes the provision of specialist local services. The situation often arises where no local service is 'ideal' for the person and there is a choice between making the best of a bad job (fitting the person into available local services) or referral to a distant specialist service (at high cost both monetarily and socially, and cutting the person off from their social network and community).

On the other hand, there are a number of people who present to physical health services, especially at the general practice level, with what are primarily mental health concerns. Here several issues can be difficult. First, there is the question of whether non-psychiatrist doctors can correctly identify mental health problems and employ the most appropriate intervention. Second, whether the individual is willing to accept that they have a mental health problem, with all the stigma that this implies. Third, whether people who experience mental health problems have their physical health problems dealt with adequately by physical healthcare services. At the level of general practice, many surgeries are relatively inaccessible to people with more serious mental health problems because of their precise surgery hours, appointment systems and waiting times. Similar difficulties exist in secondary physical healthcare, and at both levels there are concerns about the way in which doctors and other health workers fail to take seriously the physical symptoms reported by people identified as having mental health problems (another manifestation of disbelieving what people with such difficulties say). These factors conspire to ensure that a substantial proportion of people with mental health difficulties have undiagnosed and untreated physical health problems (Ananth, 1984; Honig et al., 1992).

Problems can also arise between mental health and other specialist services, for example those for people with learning disabilities and those for older people. Clearly, the principle is that no-one should, by virtue of their mental health problems, be denied the specialist input of a physical health service or a service for people with learning disabilities or a service for older people (or vice versa). However, the reality is often considerably more complex with all manner of demarcation disputes and disagreements. The major danger is of people with multiple problems being shuffled between different services, falling between the cracks and otherwise failing to get the support they need.

Local circumstances and structures are likely to determine the balance between different services, but some forum for arbitration of disputes is vital if multiply disabled people are not to be additionally disadvantaged. There must also be some spirit of compromise. There will never be a service that is ideal for everyone but, with a little creativity, bending of the 'custom and practice' (rules) of services and tailoring of resources around the individual, it is often possible to provide at least an adequate service for those people for whom a particular set of facilities were not specifically intended.

Who defines priorities?

In order to determine priorities, decisions must be made about whose needs should take precedence and under what circumstances. Such complex considerations are aggravated and proper debate stifled by the fact that because of their political sensitivity, specific priority criteria are often more implicit than explicit. There appears to be a desire to perpetuate the myth that the British National Health Service treats all comers with all problems. When health services make statements about limited resources and prioritization the resulting media attention tends to cast governing politicians in an unfavourable light (Crail, 1997). Nevertheless, if the services a person receives are not to be a simple accident of geography or the whim of individual clinicians – even within a single district different teams can have different policies – then it is important to explicitly discuss and debate prioritization criteria.

Decisions concerning who should receive help and who should not may be informed by clinical expertise (for example, research demonstrating the effectiveness of different interventions) but they are not, in the final analysis, clinical decisions. The choice of, for example, helping someone who has serious disabilities and a diagnosis of schizophrenia and someone who is experiencing acute distress following a rape – distress that, because of the recent nature of the event, has not yet become either enduring or seriously disabling – is in the end an ethical or political judgement.

As we have already discussed in the Introduction, different stakeholders have conflicting views about mental healthcare and they also have conflicting views about the prioritization of services. Arbitrating between these different views is primarily an ethical/political exercise, yet it is clinicians who must make priority judgements in relation to individuals referred to them. On a day-to-day basis the individual clinical team must decide who they should prioritize and who they should not, often on the basis of broad policy guidelines that may have contradictory implications and allow considerable room for latitude and individual judgement. Even if one places primary emphasis on the demands for help of service users themselves, this does not solve the difficulties facing clinicians as some people are clearly in a better position to make their demands heard than others. In general it is, by definition, those who are least socially disabled by their mental health problems who are in the best position to make their demands heard precisely because of their greater social abilities: he or she who shouts the loudest, and shouts in the right place and to the right people, is not always the most in need of support and help. In addition those who are discriminated against because of race, age, gender, class and disability are also less likely to have their voices heard.

In absolute terms, many people have needs that mental health services may be able to meet but given limited resources such absolutes do not apply. Instead, relative judgements must be made all the time. Typically, the question facing a clinician is whether the needs of a new referral are greater than those of an existing service user. Of course relative judgements can be made that change the capacity of a service. Every professional must balance size of caseload and amount of input to individuals on that caseload. Is it better to take on an extra person and reduce input to the remainder? And how far can this go before the input is so low that there is little point in having a caseload at all? If you only see a CPN once a year is it worth having a CPN?

There are no absolute right or wrong answers concerning who should be served by mental health services. There are policy statements to guide clinicians, but often these are somewhat vague and contradictory. For example, there is a desire to establish a primary care-led NHS (DoH, 1996) yet the priorities of GPs on mental health services are typically at odds with those of health authorities and other agencies. There is a desire to provide user-oriented care (Campbell, 1997) yet equal priority is placed on public safety and compulsion that is at odds with the wishes of individual service recipients. There is a desire to ensure a separation of 'health' and 'social' care but little guidance around the numerous demarcation disputes that inevitably arise.

4

'Severe mental illness': the problems of prioritization

British mental health policy explicitly states that efforts and resources should be focused on those people who have 'severe mental illness'. While for policy-makers the need is defined in terms of the severity of mental health problems, the different interest groups – service users themselves, the courts, professionals, relatives, neighbours – will prioritize different aspects of need. The policy statements which demand prioritization of those with 'severe mental illness' do not go on to detail how this might be achieved. Instead, some offer a series of dimensions which should be considered (DoH, 1993b; 1995a). Based on work and practice from several sources (Bachrach, 1988a; Powell and Slade, 1995) three key elements are identified – diagnosis, disability and duration – with the addition of two further dimensions *which have secured widespread acceptance at a local level* (DoH, 1995a): 'safety' and 'informal or formal care'.

While this approach offers guidance about the variables that should be considered, it hardly offers criteria for prioritization. The precise guidelines for inclusion or exclusion on each dimension are not specified. How disabled does a person have to be? Which diagnoses should be included? Further, the precedence accorded each of the dimensions is not clear. Must a person have difficulties on all dimensions? If so, someone who is profoundly disabled but presents no safety risk would not be prioritized. If a person requires difficulties on only some of the dimensions, which ones would be considered necessary? Could someone who posed a serious risk of violence to others but manifested no disabilities and had no psychiatric diagnosis receive priority mental healthcare? The implications of each of these dimensions need careful consideration before they are used as a criteria for prioritization.

Safety

The criterion of safety encompasses both the safety of the individual service user and the safety of other people. It covers both 'unintentional' harm such as self-neglect, more active self-harm, harm to other people and harm by other people: physical, sexual, emotional or financial abuse (DoH, 1995a). Clearly, safety is important but judgements in this area are fraught with problems about what constitutes 'acceptable risk'. While someone with dementia wandering off and getting lost on a cold night is clearly in danger, the position is less clear for someone who tried to kill herself the last time she lived in a flat on her own, 20 years ago, and has now returned to independent living.

The difficult balance between the rights of the individual to live as they wish and the duty of care of professionals is further confused by a duty on professionals to protect other people – the public. Such judgements necessarily involve risk-taking – the rights of the individual *versus* public comfort and safety – and in the view of many clinicians the scales are heavily weighted in favour of caution in this regard. Newspaper articles proclaiming the way in which people have been assisted to live more independently outside hospital are very few and far between. Headlines which explain how clinicians carelessly allowed someone out of hospital to harm someone else (or themselves) are disturbingly common despite the relative rarity of such events.

The extremely biased press coverage of mental health issues both seriously damages the lives of many thousands of people living with serious mental health problems by terrifying the general public, and obscures the need for better community support services by prescribing incarceration as the only solution. In reality, it has been estimated that in England approximately 20 murders per year are committed by people known to have mental health problems (Royal College of Psychiatrists, 1996), each of which receives major headlines and an expensive and protracted inquiry. The remaining 220 000 people with a diagnosis of schizophrenia estimated to be living in England and Wales (CSAG, 1995) receive little or no press coverage. It is not known what positive contribution these people make to the communities in which they live. This is not considered newsworthy.

Informal and formal care

It is clearly the case that a person with mental health problems may have a relatively high level of social functioning which is only achieved because of the level of support they are receiving. This care criterion encompasses both the help that a person receives from relatives, friends and other informal networks as well as that from formal services, paid staff and hospital or residential facilities. Additionally, however, this criterion covers detention under the Mental Health Act. If it has been deemed necessary to compulsorily detain someone then the input that they must receive is, at least in part, specified within the Act and priority must be given to this formal care.

This area poses several dilemmas for clinicians. First, because of the requirement to prioritize those people who are subject to detention under the Mental Health Act and ensure their subsequent aftercare, this may lead to a skewing of mental health resources towards the compulsory end of the spectrum. It may be possible to obviate the need for compulsion if resources are available for the ongoing support, respite and early preventative work to avoid the crisis that may lead to compulsory detention. However, if a disproportionate amount of resource is tied up in compulsory detention and its sequelae, then these preventative measures may become less possible and a vicious circle established with more compulsory detentions leading to more resources being allocated to this area. If inpatient resources are scarce then a clinical team can defer, maybe indefinitely, the admission of a voluntary patient or discharge them prematurely. Thus the needs of those people who seek help voluntarily take second place, probably at considerable cost to the individuals involved.

Second, if a person is functioning well with a given amount of support from formal and informal carers, including the treatment/medication they provide, it is often difficult to ascertain whether this amount of support continues to be necessary. It is possible that, after a period of time, a person may develop the resources to manage more independently but it is very difficult to test this. Memories of past crises and fears of precipitating future difficulties mean that clinicians, informal carers and sometimes users themselves are often fearful of 'rocking the boat' and experimenting with moves towards greater independence. Additionally, clinicians may be motivated to keep known and able users within their services rather than enabling them to move on thereby risking taking on less able and more 'difficult' newcomers. It is, after all, a bonus to have good workers in a sheltered workshop, even if they could obtain open employment, or people who help with household chores in a hostel, even if they could manage in a place of their own.

The over-provision of care and support is not only wasteful of scarce resources, but more importantly it further disables, by de-skilling, already disabled people. Many disabled people lack confidence in their abilities and therefore may fail to make the most of their lives. If they are to develop the confidence necessary to do the things they want to do then they need others – clinicians, friends, relatives and neighbours – to have confidence in them. It is very difficult to believe in yourself if everyone around you doubts you. While it is clearly damaging to withdraw support and help that continues to be necessary, it is equally important to work with service users to enable them to take the risks to grow and develop. While research evidence may be able to guide such judgements of 'risk', it cannot make them. On the one hand it is not always available and on the other, based as it is on populations, it is impossible to tell whether or not the individual will be typical of the research population examined.

Finally, consideration of the amount of formal and informal support a person is receiving may result in under-provision of care. If someone is receiving a particular, relatively low, level of input and functioning adequately, then it is easy to assume that additional support would not convey any great advantage. For example, it is often implicitly or explicitly assumed that the 'negative symptoms' of schizophrenia are a necessary consequence of an assumed disease process, even though the work of Wing and Brown (1970) clearly showed that the social situation in which people are placed, and the input that they receive, can markedly change their extent.

Diagnosis

According to *Building Bridges* (DoH, 1995a), diagnosis *may* include psychotic illness, dementia, severe neurotic illness, personality disorder or developmental disorder. As such the diagnostic criterion is very broadly drawn – however, it should also be noted that the term 'may' is included as opposed to something more directive like 'will' or 'should'. This means that there is scope for individual interpretation and inconsistency. While there would probably be little disagreement concerning 'psychotic illnesses' this may not be the case for people with neurotic problems even though someone with, say, severe obsessive compulsive disorder may be considerably more disabled than someone with a psychosis. As Barker (1997) suggests:

'It is probably accurate to say that many now assume that SEMI [serious and enduring mental illness] often means schizophrenia. The obvious implication is that all other mental health problems are 'minor' or non-serious in nature. The major irony of the emerging narrowing of the definition of SEMI is the potential for adding insult to the psychic injury of sufferers from depression of classifying them, inadvertently, as part of the so-called 'worried well'.

For people with a diagnosis of personality disorder, the problem is not one of 'psychic injury' but of being considered ineligible for services. Many services reject those people whose primary diagnosis is one of personality disorder, and some of those people for whom this is a secondary diagnosis depending upon the nature of their problems:

'When the service user does not "fit" the narrow bands of labels defined as "illness" or is difficult or disliked, there is an assignment of the usual dustbin diagnosis "personality disorder". The personality disorder categories are therapeutic death. Clinical euphemisms for "I don't know" and "I don't want to know." (Pembroke, 1997)

Typically, there is a desire to withdraw service from those who are the most disruptive, disturbing and difficult to help: those who upset other service users, make demands on services that are considered excessive or inappropriate and lack any apparent desire to change (Bachrach, 1989; Hirsch *et al.*, 1992; Repper and Perkins, 1994). It often appears that people manifesting behaviours such as these receive diagnoses like 'personality disorder' or 'alcohol/drug misuse' and that these are used as a way of withdrawing service either through discharge or through the setting of contracts that the person cannot or will not meet (Perkins and Repper, 1996).

Clinicians may assert that 'we cannot help' or 'we have nothing to offer them' or 'they are not mentally ill'. Ironically, it remains the case that while people can be rejected from and discharged by services because they have personality disorders and are 'not mentally ill', they can at the same time be compulsorily detained in those services under the 1983 Mental Health Act within which 'personality disorder' is explicitly included. This can lead to the somewhat bizarre situation of people being alternately compulsorily detained within and excluded from mental health services (Perkins and Repper, 1996). Although mental health services are often ambivalent about helping this group of people, this does not mean that their problems disappear. Instead, they may be taken to other agencies – social services, housing, voluntary and informal community services – who often feel they lack the expertise to provide support. When such agencies look to health services for assistance they too often find them reluctant to help: they deem the individual not to have mental health problems and therefore to be outside their remit. Not only does this sour relationships between different agencies but, more importantly, it means that the individual in distress fails to get the help they need. It often appears to be the case that there is a difference between popular and professional definitions of madness in this regard. There are a group of distressed, disabled and 'disruptive' individuals whom professionals deem not to be mentally ill but whose behaviour is construed by local communities and non-mental health agencies to be indicative of madness.

Research literature has demonstrated on numerous occasions that diagnosis in psychiatry is not a precise science: agreement between skilled clinicians concerning diagnosis is relatively low (Bentall, 1990). Similarly, diagnosis is not a good predictor of prognosis, hospitalization, response to treatment or level of disability (Birley, 1991; Bentall *et al.*, 1988). It is therefore unfortunately the case that diagnostic criteria, while superficially attractive, are necessarily problematic as a criterion for determining the relative need of different individuals. In this context, level of disability may be a more important yardstick.

Disability

As outlined in *Building Bridges* (DoH, 1995a), the disability criterion of severity of mental health problems refers to a person's ability to function in the community. In particular, employment, recreation, personal care, domestic and personal relationship arenas are cited. Ideas about disability in relation to mental health problems have a long history in British psychiatry (Wing and Morris, 1981). It has been argued that the aim of mental health services in working with people who experience serious ongoing mental health problems should be to minimize the socially disabling impact of these problems by ensuring that the person has access to the ordinary roles, relationships, activities and opportunities that they desire (Perkins and Repper, 1996).

While a social disability and access perspective may be a useful organizing principle for services, it can pose dilemmas for clinicians in terms of prioritization. If the most disabled people are to be prioritized then resources will tend not to be allocated to the prevention of disability. Rather than preserving a person's social functioning there will be a tendency to wait until it has deteriorated to the point where resource allocation is warranted. As it is generally easier to maintain something than re-establish it when it is lost, this may both increase disability unnecessarily and be wasteful of resources.

Most disability theorists would argue that the extent of a person's disability is largely socially determined (Perkins and Repper, 1996). For example, Wing and Morris (1981) define social disadvantages as one of three key contributors to the extent of a person's disability. These include both those disadvantages that pre-date the individual's mental health problems and thus influence the resources they have to cope with these problems when they occur (disrupted family relationships, poor education, unemployment, poverty), and those which are a consequence of their mental health problems (unemployment, limited social network, poverty, poor housing, discrimination, rejection by family/friends). If extent of disability is used as a major prioritization criterion then suffering may be unnecessarily increased by a person having to lose their job, friends and home before they can get help rather than receiving support to maintain these in the first place. Furthermore, there may be a danger of deploying health resources to compensate for social inequalities: mental health services will never be a substitute for employment, an adequate income, decent housing, a proper education and the social inclusion that goes along with these.

There may be some types of difficulties that take precedence over others. If, for example, an individual's interpersonal relationship problems mean that they are disruptive in the community, then these needs are likely to take priority over those of someone whose disabilities are at least as problematic to them but less problematic to others. For example, a person who rarely goes out, has no friends, no job, no leisure pursuits but does not disturb the neighbours, is likely to receive lower priority than the person who is disruptive, disturbs the neighbours at night and engages in petty thieving.

There may be other areas in which different disabilities might receive different priority depending upon individual and social circumstances. For example, support with employment may be viewed as more important for someone who has had a good job and lost it as a consequence of their mental health problems than for someone who was excluded from school in his early teens, whose literacy is poor and who has never worked. Alternatively, the poor self-care and attention to domestic matters of someone living in an upmarket area of town may be a matter of greater concern than that of someone living in a more run-down area. Factors such as these can skew the judgements of the clinicians required to decide upon relative disability and need, and once again different stakeholders will have different views about the priority of different disabilities.

Duration

If priority is to be accorded to those people with enduring mental health problems then some criterion relating to the longevity of difficulties is necessary. However, *Building Bridges* (DoH, 1995a) is somewhat vague in this regard:

'periods which vary between six months and more than two years'.

The main difficulty with a longevity criterion in prioritization is that it may, in itself, tend to be the cause of long-term problems. There is evidence of a relationship between the (longer) duration of untreated problems prior to first episode, and the subsequent (increased) probability of relapse (Macmillan *et al.*, 1986). This, combined with evidence that every relapse increases the possibility of future crises and tends to result in increased social disability (Hogarty *et al.*, 1991), suggests that intensive input and support at the start of a period of problems could substantially decrease the development of disability and the consequent need for long-term support. Waiting until a person has had difficulties for long enough to warrant prioritization may mean, for example, that their social networks and family relationships become more damaged, that they lose their job, and that their self-confidence is unnecessarily eroded. Repairing the damage done may be difficult, and would almost certainly take more input and resource than preventing the damage in the first place.

Wants, motivation and the likelihood of success

Although those people with 'severe mental illness' are the designated priority group for mental health services, in allocating scarce resources it is often tempting for clinicians to adopt additional criteria in determining the amount of effort to expend with different people. It is important that any discussion of priorities – who should be served – include not only explicit policy but actual practice. In this context there are a number of implicit factors which, even if they do not influence who is seen, often determine the optimism and commitment of the clinician and the amount of effort that is put into the work.

A user's desire for help can have an important influence on the service they receive. Clearly, those people who are compulsorily detained must receive priority in inpatient facilities. However, for all of those who are not compulsorily engaged with services, clinicians usually (and understandably) prefer to work with someone who actively wants our input than with someone who rejects it every step of the way or is critical of what we do.

It will always be difficult at an individual level for clinicians to prioritize and expend time and energy with people who do not want or appreciate their help. Not only do people who are reluctant to receive support evoke questions about how, whether and what support should be provided, but it may be tempting to devote more resources to those who are more welcoming of our attention. However, this is problematic for two reasons. First, those who are not grateful for assistance may be very disabled and in need of support. Given the prejudice against people with mental health problems, it is understandable why many will not welcome the input of mental health practitioners and services and will not want to need help. Second, many of those who do not want help retain a great many characteristics that would, in someone without mental health problems, be considered positive: pride, determination, ordinary expectations and ambitions (Thompson, 1988). Their reluctance to need assistance may in fact be a manifestation of a desirable independence that is lacking among some of those who lack confidence in their abilities and welcome professional support. The onus is not, however, on people with mental health problems to avail themselves of whatever services are on offer, but on services to render themselves accessible, acceptable and able to meet the particular needs of even the most reluctant.

A related factor revolves around users' apparent 'motivation to change'. Once again, clinicians often prefer to invest time and energy in someone who appears to use their input as it is intended to be used, rather than in someone who appears not to want to change and seems to 'abuse' that which is offered. Sometimes it is tempting to use 'contracts' which specify the conditions for using services as a way of excluding such people if they do not adhere to the rules (Perkins and Repper, 1996).

The dilemmas facing clinicians in this regard generally revolve around differences concerning who is right. When clinicians talk about 'motivation to change' this generally means that the user shares the clinician's immediate goals and does what the clinician thinks they ought to do in order to achieve these. If clinician and user differ about goals, or the ways in which these should be achieved, then problems arise. The clinician must balance the adoption of a user-centred approach, acceding to the user's wishes where this is possible, and continuing to insist on what they firmly believe to be best.

There are also issues of 'treatability' and the likely 'success' of input. Although policy states that priority should be accorded to those who have the most severe problems, there is an understandable pull in a different direction towards allocating resources to those people with more 'treatable' problems where 'success' is more likely. If resources are scarce it is not unreasonable to argue that they should be used where they are likely to have most effect. In considering such dilemmas, ideas about relative success also need to be examined. For example, which represents greater success: a man with a diagnosis of schizophrenia who had been hospitalized for

10 years now successfully living in his own flat (although still unemployed and heavily dependent on services), or a man who lost his job as a consequence of a time-limited period of depression regaining employment and being discharged from services completely? If success is seen solely in terms of cessation of service usage – discharge – then the latter would be prioritized. If success is viewed more in terms of quality of life then the position would be different.

Most clinicians have been trained in a variety of cure-based models, via whatever means – medication, psychotherapy, family therapy, counselling – removing a person's problems so that they cease to need help. The reality of services prioritizing those who have the most serious mental health problems is that such cure-based approaches are inappropriate (Ekdawi and Conning, 1994; Perkins and Repper, 1996): if clinicians' motivation remains rooted in ideas of cure and discharge then problems will arise.

A need for criteria?

In a search for clarity there is often a wish to devise specific and fixed criteria for acceptance into a service. However, this can be intensely problematic. It can almost be guaranteed that the criteria adopted by each support agency will leave gaps meaning that some people will fail to get the services they need. The problem of people 'falling through the cracks' between services is well documented (Clifford et al., 1988; Repper and Perkins, 1995). If this is to be avoided then good communication among clinicians and agencies on the ground, at a local level, is critical. There needs to be explicit consideration of who is best placed to serve whom, together with an acceptance that a proportion of users will fall outside the remit of all organizations and a commitment to negotiation to ensure that such people do receive the help that they need.

Instead of the set criteria for acceptance that may create cracks, it is probably preferable that each agency specifies their 'core business': the core group of people for whom they are designed and the specific skills they have at their disposal. Between the core business of different agencies there can then be flexibility and negotiation about who is best placed to serve each person whose problems do not fall within the core remit of any group.

If some people are to receive no service at all, or only a limited portion of resources, then this must be made explicit and agreed so that individual clinicians are not blamed every time someone fails to receive a service. A delicate balance must be struck between trying to serve all comers (and serving no-one well), and offering an impeccable service to only a small proportion of those who need it. Once again, this balance may be informed by clinicians, but it involves essentially political choices about the standards of service that citizens can expect. The various Patient's Charters (DoH, 1993a) represent an attempt to grapple with this issue, but at present they are typically vague in most important areas and the trade-off between offering particular stand-ards and the capacity of the service has not been explicitly addressed. Until such dif-ficult issues have been considered, the dilemmas facing clinicians will be exacerbated.

Finally, any discussion of service criteria and prioritization is predicated on the assumption that it is necessary to restrict entry. In reality, mental health services increasingly face the problems not of excluding potential users, but of including and engaging those who are considered to need help but are reluctant to accept it. Issues of the accessibility, acceptability and appropriateness of services to the people who need them are central. If services are unattractive, inaccessible because of prejudice or culture or geography and seen as failing to provide what people with mental health problems see themselves as needing, then many people who could benefit from, and should receive, support will fail to do so, irrespective of criteria set for the provision of services.

5

Rights, protection
and duty of care

Any society places limits on the behaviour of its citizens. These limits act primarily when a person makes choices which interfere with the rights of others. At their most extreme, these limits, and the consequences of contravening them, are enshrined in the laws of the society. It is typically held that a society's laws apply equally to all citizens but there are exceptions, most notably when a person is considered to have mental health problems. Thus, when a person is deemed to be 'mentally incompetent' there exists a special set of laws just for them which appear in mental health legislation. Such legislation permits, under certain circumstances, an individual's preferences and rights to be over-ridden by psychiatric services. It allows compulsory detention and treatment of an individual against their will – actions that are only permissible if the individual is considered to have mental health problems.

There may be many justifications for such an inequality. It is very hard to stand by and watch someone do something that one believes to be profoundly detrimental, even life-threatening, when one has a means of preventing the difficulties. However, the existence of special 'mental health' legislation means that those who experience cognitive and emotional problems are not treated in the same way as other citizens and do not have the rights of other citizens. The inequalities are particularly stark when a parallel is drawn with physical health problems. A person with a life-threatening physical condition has the right to refuse treatment for that condition, even if there are interventions which all available evidence suggests would be effective in treating it. The existence of special mental health legislation means that someone who is deemed to have serious mental health difficulties does not enjoy such rights and can be compulsorily treated against their will.

Yet it is the belief in the physical causes of some 'mental illness' that has been used to justify involuntary detention and treatment. If a person's loss of competency (as defined by others) is deemed to be biologically determined, then treatment – even against their will – is a rational means of restoring competency. As Sherlock (1986) argues:

'On the one hand we are more sensitive than ever to claims patients make for their autonomy while at the same time our understanding of the biological roots of their illness may afford us powerful tools with which to treat them even in the absence of their consent. Even where such tools are absent, a biological understanding of mental disease orients us to the way that serious mental disorder incapacitates the person against his or her own will and may require care and custody even in the absence of cure.'

Mental health professionals are caught between on the one hand a legal framework and professional codes of conduct which impose upon them a 'duty of care' and a requirement to help people in distress 'for their own good', and on the other hand the expressed wishes, demands and rights of these people. Such contradictory expectations of professionals show no signs of abating. Exhortations to provide services that accord with the wishes and preferences of users are increasing (Bowl, 1996; Campbell, 1997) **but at the same time** demands to protect the public and disabled individuals themselves are escalating (Zito Trust, 1995; *Panorama*, 1997). In such a climate, clinicians cannot avoid the ethical dilemmas imposed by conflicts between duty of care and civil rights. It is important to consider the implications of both so that informed decisions can be made. It is not enough to follow blindly the path of well-meaning paternalism, or maternalism, so prevalent in many services.

An uncompromising 'duty of care' perspective

A 'duty of care' perspective starts from the premise that a society, via its clinicians, has an obligation to provide support and treatment for those who have serious mental health problems: to protect vulnerable people from the folly of their own misguided judgements. Such an approach is predicated on the belief that people with mental health problems cannot make sound judgements about what they need and want. It is assumed that those very mental processes – the processes of emotion and cognition – that are required to make appropriate judgements have malfunctioned.

This type of analysis has two major implications. First, it would be irresponsible and unethical to allow people with mental health problems to do what they want. Their cognitive and emotional difficulties prevent them from really knowing what they want or what is good for them, so someone else must make decisions for them. Second, it would be unethical to hold someone with mental health problems responsible for their actions. Their cognitive and emotional difficulties mean that they are not responsible for what they do.

Clearly, it is often the case that people with mental health problems will do as they are told by clinicians or other carers. It is important to recognize that a great deal done by clinicians 'for someone's own good' is not performed under the auspices of legislation. Rewards for compliance, such as the approval of staff, verbal persuasion, argument and giving or withdrawing attention are at least as important (Perkins, 1996b). However, in order to ensure that people can be required to do that which is deemed to be good for them, a legislative framework exists, as a bottom line, to permit compulsion.

One consequence of a 'duty of care' perspective is provision for forced detention and treatment when it is considered that a person cannot make decisions for themselves. If someone will not accept the treatment that clinicians consider would be good for them then they can be forcibly treated. The existence of such legislation offers an important 'back-up threat' in ensuring that service users do what clinicians dictate: 'If you do not do this then you will be sectioned'. As Campbell (1996b) describes, it is the knowledge that treatment can be enforced, as much as the actual enforcing of it, that effectively strips users of power.

A second consequence involves excusing people with serious mental health problems from criminal responsibility for their actions. This is reflected in a variety of 'diversion from custody' schemes and alternatives to prison for people who have mental health problems. Usually such absolution is partial – the mental health problems contributed to their criminal behaviour but did not wholly account for it. However, this is a compromise. Within an 'uncompromising' duty of care perspective where it is assumed that a person with serious mental health problems cannot make decisions about what is best for them, it stands to reason that they cannot be held criminally responsible for their decisions and behaviour.

This type of perspective has the advantage of absolving individuals from responsibilities that they may not be in a position to take. It also enables people to receive support and help when they may not be in a position to determine their needs. However, this is all achieved at the expense of their rights as a citizen, their rights to make decisions about their life and how they wish to live it. The idea that someone might have choices is obviated if it is considered that a person's cognitive problems mean that they lack the ability to make effective judgements. If someone is deemed mad, their wishes and decisions must be faulty (except in so far as they agree with the clinician's), are a symptom of their mental health problems, and can therefore be discounted.

An uncompromising individual 'civil rights' perspective

The denial of the rights of people with serious mental health problems that is inherent in a 'duty of care' approach and the horrors of forced treatment have been of concern to many, particularly those in the mental health user/survivor movement (Campbell, 1996a; Chamberlin, 1984, 1990). However, probably the prime exponent of a pure 'civil rights' perspective is the mental health system survivor and lawyer Ron Thompson, who was the Washington DC representative of the US National Association of Psychiatric Survivors. Thompson (1993a) is extremely critical of the *legal doctrine and bedrock professional practice of forced treatment*:

'the right of degreed professionals… to force dangerous drugs/"medications" on persons who are not allowed by law to defend themselves, and to tell themselves, their patient/inmates, and the world at large, that they are doing this for the good of those individuals.'

In analysing speeches made by President Clinton in which it is suggested there can be no legitimate rationale for distinguishing between 'mental' and 'physical' illnesses in areas like research, insurance and individual entitlement, Thompson argues that such a perspective clearly ignores the fact that many mentally ill persons cannot, by law, refuse treatment (Thompson, 1993c). He comments that there must be:

'something wrong with the situation that the problems of the least clearly and most elusively (or non-existent) physical nature had nevertheless permitted psychiatrists a power undreamed of by doctors engaged in the treatment of clearly biological illnesses.' (Thompson, 1993d)

The essence of Thompson's (1993d) argument is that the mental health system is based on three premises:

1 the biochemical nature of mental illness
2 the need for forced treatment
3 the excusing or denial of personal responsibility for acts otherwise against the law.

'[This] iron triangle of bio-coercive psychiatry… add[s] up not to a health care system but to a remarkable and ingenious shell game in which all three ideas are either morally or factually wrong, but because of the relationships between them, each appears to be supported by the other two… The purpose of this giant house of cards is not to provide medical care, but to allow all parties to it (including many of the willing patients) a feeling of control over these problems, and at the same time the avoidance of an uncomfortable conscience if the real purpose of the system was admitted to themselves and the world.' (Thompson, 1993d)

Thompson (1993a, 1993b, 1993c, 1993d) argues that the need for forced treatment is justified on the basis that mental 'illnesses' – dysfunctional thoughts and emotions – result from endogenous brain biochemical or gene malfunctions. These mean that the person cannot be held responsible for what they do. If they cannot be accountable for what they do because of their brain problems, others must decide and forced treatment is therefore justifiable. Each of the elements – the biochemical nature of problems, the denial of personal responsibility and forced treatment – are interrelated and mutually justify the other premises.

Thompson argues that if cognitive and emotional problems did not derive from endogenous biochemical or genetic problems but were instead a consequence of life histories, abuse, the absence of caring adults etc., then the system would break down – but this is not necessarily the case. It would be entirely possible to argue that the consequences of abuse, neglect and adversity render a person unable to make decisions for themselves and thus allow the continuance of compulsory treatment. The stronger element in Thompson's analysis is the link between excusing and/or denying personal responsibility to those deemed to have mental health problems and the licence which this gives to professionals to do things against a person's will including enforced treatment and the prevention of self-harm.

The individual civil rights perspective adopted by Thompson takes the position that it is morally wrong to deny those with mental health problems responsibility for their behaviour. This means, on the one hand, that forced treatment can never be justified but on the other that someone with cognitive/emotional problems who breaks the law is accountable for their behaviour in the same way as anyone else. He draws upon the 'educational' films produced in Germany in the mid-1930s designed to:

'accustom various professional groups and university students to the "release" (i.e. murder) of mental patients from their "useless lives"... the narrator soothingly said that these individuals would undoubtedly wish to be "released" from their "useless lives" if they were not so sick that they were unable to ask for this kindness and consideration on their own.' (Thompson, 1993c)

Thompson points out that the arguments which allowed 300 000 mental patients to be killed in Germany adopted:

'exactly the same rationale, and in exactly the same tones, which is always given for involuntary [psychiatric] *treatment.'* (Thompson, 1993c)

There are a number of people in the user/survivor movement who believe that the consequences of not adopting this pure civil rights position are too serious, in terms of denial of personhood and withdrawal of rights to define one's own interests. For the benefits of no forced treatment and the right to receive support and help on their own terms, they are prepared to accept the fact that some people may sometimes make ill-advised decisions that have consequences detrimental to them (Thompson, 1993a, 1993b, 1993c, 1993d). If this position is adopted, then many of the problems concerning the relative importance accorded to the views of different stakeholders evaporate. At the bottom line it is up to the person with mental health problems to determine what they want or need, for providers to furnish this within the resources that can be secured, and for society to operate the same constraints on people with mental health problems as it does on any citizen.

The grey area of compromise

Between an uncompromising individual civil rights perspective and a total duty of care approach, most would probably wish to adopt some form of compromise. While care may be important, few would really be prepared to adopt a totally paternalistic stand and completely deny the agency and citizenship of those with mental health problems. Likewise while civil rights are important, few would be prepared to hold someone who is extremely distressed and disturbed fully responsible for their behaviour at all times.

In considering an appropriate compromise between civil rights and duty of care it would be possible to start from either end. It would be possible to start from the assumption that people with mental health problems need to be protected and then decide which individuals could make decisions for themselves, and within which constraints. Alternatively, it would be possible to start from the view that each individual has the right to make decisions for themselves and to bear the consequences of these decisions, and then consider where compromises might be desirable.

It is certainly the case that people with serious mental health problems have been, and continue to be, denied their rights as citizens: denied access to the roles, relationships, facilities, activities and opportunities in society that those who are not so disabled enjoy (Perkins and Repper, 1996). This has been recognized in both the Americans with Disabilities Act (1993) and the UK Disability Discrimination Act (1995); both pieces of civil rights legislation designed to improve access for those with disabilities, including those resulting from mental health problems. It is equally the case that within mental health services themselves, the voice and rights of those who use them have historically been ignored. Extensive user action over the last decade has begun to reverse this trend (Barker and Peck, 1996; Campbell, 1996b) but there is still a long way to go. As the oppression of people who experience serious mental health problems will undoubtedly continue until they enjoy full rights as citizens, we feel it is important to *start* from a civil rights perspective.

From an uncompromising civil rights standpoint, everyone with mental health problems has the same rights and responsibilities as anyone else. Forced treatment is never justified and actions can never be excused because of mental health difficulties. In this way, Thompson's (1993c) very individualistic analysis makes clear links between rights and responsibilities: a person cannot have the rights of a citizen unless they are also able to accept the responsibilities placed on all citizens. Many others who are equally concerned with the rights of those with mental health problems (*see* Chamberlin, 1990) do not share such an individual view or place such parallel emphasis on responsibilities. In this context the existing legal system makes provision for 'mitigating circumstances' to be taken into account. It seems not unreasonable that some of this mitigation might apply to those whose reality is profoundly different from that of others. Having been beaten counts as mitigation for attacking someone. Therefore could not believing that one has been attacked or abused (even if this is seen as 'delusional') equally be seen as a mitigating circumstance, and thus grounds for decreasing (but not removing completely) the person's responsibility for their act? It seems reasonable to assume that individuals act and make moral judgements about the world on the basis of their beliefs or constructions about the world. For some people with mental health problems, these constructions are shared by no-one else. Therefore questions concerning the extent of their responsibility for actions in the world as others see it may be open to question.

One difficulty with a purely individual civil rights perspective is that it omits any notion of the collective responsibility that a society may have for its more vulnerable members (Sayce, 1998). Such a collective responsibility means entering the grey area of what members of a society can expect of each other. Clearly this is relevant in relation to access and inclusion in communities and the provision of support and help to make this possible, but it is also relevant in relation to intervening when a person is in distress. Many might find it unacceptable to imagine a society in which people would stand by and watch someone kill him/herself or live in squalor, and if such things are to be avoided then it may occasionally be necessary to act against a person's will. For example, the authors know a woman who is eternally grateful to a stranger who asked her to come down from the parapet of a bridge from which she had decided to jump and when she did not, pulled her off and insisted on walking her home: a variant of 'forced treatment'.

Compulsory detention and treatment

Clearly, compulsory treatment is only necessary when a person does not agree with that which professionals consider necessary. In view of the potentially destructive consequences of compulsion it must only be used when there are no alternatives: the negative effects on the individual's self-concept, their trust in services, their relationship with the staff members involved and their role and relationships within their family, the inevitable stigma attached to being sectioned and the implications of this for management within services ('they needed to be sectioned last time') and the interpretation of a history of involuntary detention by employers and colleagues. In this regard there are a number of questions which clinicians must ask.

Who should decide?

At present the law makes provision for mental health professionals to determine what should be done and how the person should be treated. However, this does not have to be the case. There have been successful pilots of the use of crisis cards in which a person makes plans in advance about what they would like to happen. The individual can then carry a copy of this on his/her person and the mental health service should maintain a copy in their notes. Such plans enable an individual to make their own decisions about what should happen to them at times when they cannot make decisions for themselves (Lindow, 1996; Bryant and McClelland, 1997). While these cards clearly cannot be used for the first crisis which a person experiences, they can be in subsequent crises. The real question is whether professionals are prepared to respect the decisions made.

For how long?

Most forced treatment in the UK greatly exceeds the immediate crisis period. The justification for extending compulsion appears to be rooted in the biological understanding of mental illness which Sherlock put forward (*see* p. 44) and which Thompson contests (*see* p. 46). If the cause of mental incompetency is biological then treatment of this biological change needs to be imposed until competency is restored. One difficulty with this perspective arises if the person cannot be restored to 'the way they were'. As Atkinson (1991) asks:

'How far can society impose its norms on that person when they are no longer appropriate? Is it not possible to allow autonomy within the new framework of the person's thinking?

Whatever the justification for continuing compulsion once a crisis has been resolved, or once the risks which that person is considered to pose have ameliorated, clinicians must explicitly consider the reasons for and against further compulsion. This introduces the question of information and informed consent. Although it may be difficult to ensure that a person understands the treatment being provided during a crisis, all too often, this assumption is made erroneously. For someone to refuse treatment they must be given information about the treatment on offer in a manner which allows them both to understand it and make their views known. Since their views may change over the period of treatment, it is also important that information is not given on a one-off basis, but that every opportunity is taken to inform the person of their legal rights, the decisions which are being made for them and the reasons for these decisions.

In this regard it is not unusual for clinicians to assume that a person can only be considered competent and rational and able to make decisions for him/herself once they agree with treatment: rational people want to be well, treatment will make them well, so a rational person will agree with treatment. However, many refuse supposedly effective treatments for physical ailments: people do have a right to refuse treatment and live in a way that others might not approve, that is their choice. The question for clinicians arises most poignantly when a person is no longer a risk but it is known that once legal obligations to be treated are removed they will cease treatment and in the past this has led to relapse. In such a situation, negotiation and compromise on the part of the clinician are probably more effective than continued insistence on a course of action the person does not want to take (Tyrer *et al.*, 1994).

In what areas?

There is a general tendency to assume that if a person cannot make decisions for him/herself in relation to one area, they cannot make them in any area and everything they say should be disregarded. This can lead to an extremely poor relationship between individual and clinician and further erode the person's confidence in their own judgements. Within the limits set by compulsory treatment, it must be acknowledged that a person has the ability and the right to make choices about, for example, when, where and how medication is administered, when and how to wash, sleep, eat and so on. Furthermore, if a person's decision in a particular area – typically with respect to hospitalization and drugs – has been over-ruled, it is more honest to acknowledge that there are indeed different perspectives that can be taken, and in this case the power relationships favour those of the clinician. This does not mean that the clinicians are right and the user is wrong, they both have reasons for their decisions but given the circumstances the law dictates that the clinician can enforce his or her judgement.

How to decide when someone should be over-ruled?

Considering the possibility of over-ruling a person's judgement is probably the most difficult area of all. Clearly, one of the most common criteria adopted is whether the individual agrees with the prescriptions of the clinicians – if they do they are considered to have insight and no compulsion is necessary. However, given the numerous different constructions of mental health problems and preferences regarding treatment options that exist among clinicians (Karasu, 1986), it seems not unreasonable that a service user may agree with one possible option but not with others or may hold a different perspective completely. The idea that there is one true model of mental health problems and one correct treatment is very difficult to sustain. Therefore, the decision might more sensibly be based on a proper individual case approach. If previous experience shows that dire consequences follow the person's chosen course of treatment there would appear to be better grounds for over-ruling their judgement than if the person has never been assisted in trying to do what they want to do.

While such questions go some way towards raising awareness of alternatives to over-ruling a person's decisions, they will be of limited value in a service which does not provide a range of different support options. If the only treatment available is hospitalization and medication then it is less likely that the person will be able to have at least some of what they want and the probability of compulsion will be increased. Some service users, for example, may prefer to have access to talking therapies or a 24-hour non-medical crisis service (Campbell, 1996c). Others may prefer more intensive support at home (Meltzer *et al.*, 1991).

Finally, there are occasions when a civil rights perspective is used as an excuse for neglect: 'It is his right/choice to have filthy clothes, live in a very dirty room, never go out … he could wash his clothes, clean his room, go out if he wanted to.' In such an instance it is often the case that the person has not been given help and support of a type, or in a manner, that is acceptable to him. Perhaps he would wear clean clothes if someone did his washing for or with him? Perhaps his room would be clean if he had a home-help? Perhaps he feels stupid because he is having difficulty doing these things? Perhaps he cannot see the point in dressing up or going out because he doesn't know anyone or there is no-one to notice or care?

In most formulations, a civil rights perspective includes the right to that help and support which is necessary to enable a person to have access to their society. A person or group that is marginalized or excluded cannot enjoy the rights of other citizens. If people have disabilities, whether these result from cognitive and emotional or physical difficulties, then help, support and adaptation of the world is necessary to ensure access.

Once again the dilemmas rest on the balance of power and since this lies so conclusively with professionals it is easier for service users to become victims than allies. In this regard, the importance of demonstrating respect for the wishes and views of users, planning ahead for crises, negotiating treatment plans which clinicians are prepared to adhere to, and building up relationships that the user finds beneficial cannot be under-estimated. If service users had more reason to trust services to listen and respond to their wishes, they might become more willing to request support to avert crises and the need for compulsion might be reduced.

The responsibilities placed upon clinicians by the current framework of mental health legislation necessarily lead to day-to-day conflicts between ensuring the rights of the individual client, acceding to their wishes and protecting both the public and the individual from their actions. Within the legal constraints that exist are numerous decisions which necessitate ethical judgements on the part of the clinician: are the consequences of permitting someone to do what they want really dire enough to warrant the draconian step of removing their rights? Clearly anyone who commits a crime risks having their liberty and rights curtailed but for people who experience mental health problems, such curtailment typically occurs before a crime has been committed in anticipation of what they might do. Such 'preventive detention' does not occur with other groups who may be considered high risk, e.g. men who regularly get drunk and beat their wives.

Moving away from daily clinical realities, the question must be raised – can it be right to maintain different laws for those who do and do not experience mental health problems?

6

Compliance or alliance?
Informed choice and the
desirability of compliance

In the literature of policy and clinical practice of community care, issues relating to compliance loom increasingly large (Haynes *et al.*, 1979; Gardner and Hill, 1994; DoH, 1994a, 1994b, 1995b; Kemp *et al.*, 1996; Sandford, 1996). Invariably concerns about compliance are associated with drugs: whether or not people with serious mental health problems comply with the medication prescriptions of their doctors; how to ensure compliance; the impact of non-compliance on their behaviour. The typical argument is summarized by Kemp *et al.* (1996):

'Given the established efficacy of neuroleptic drugs in psychotic disorders, and the potentially devastating consequences of relapse, non-compliance is one of the major preventable causes of psychiatric morbidity and a research priority for the NHS.'

Estimated rates of non-compliance with prescribed medication vary from around 35% (Mann, 1986) to as high as 80% (Corrigan *et al.*, 1990). It has been claimed that non-compliance is associated with 43% of admissions to psychiatric hospitals (Kent and Yellowlees, 1994), and an estimated cost of around £100m per year in the UK (Davis and Drummond, 1990). Such figures have resulted in a variety of attempts to increase compliance with medication which often show little regard for the rights and choices of people who are prescribed drugs.

Attempts to increase compliance

One of the most widely discussed ways of attempting to increase psychiatric patients' compliance with medication has been the use of force. Clearly, the Mental Health Act has always allowed forced treatment within psychiatric hospitals. However, as the number of acute beds for people with mental health problems has decreased, so the number of people who can be directly subject to such powers has decreased. This situation has led to calls for legislation to allow some psychiatric patients to receive enforced treatment in the community (Royal College of Psychiatrists, 1993b). Legislation has been passed allowing 'discharge under supervision' (DoH, 1994a) – the enforced access to and supervision of some patients in the community – but sustained opposition from service user groups and other interested parties (MIND, 1993; Bynoe, 1993) has ensured that, as yet, this falls short of compulsory community treatment. The legislation does, however, increase psychiatry's powers outside hospital as illustrated by the following press release:

'A Community Supervision Order would apply to a small group of patients who are repeatedly admitted to Hospital under Detention Orders... of the Mental Health Act, and who require long term support and supervision in the Community, but are known to have a history of defaulting or failing to take their treatment. By placing them on a Community Supervision Order, the responsible medical officer would ensure their agreement [sic] to take treatment and be cared for and supervised by a care team in the community. If the patient fails to take his/her treatment and begins to deteriorate, the Order would give the responsible medical officer the power to take the patient back to hospital in order to re-establish treatment. This would ensure the patient's freedom [sic] to remain within the community and his or her right [sic] to treatment.' (Royal College of Psychiatrists, 1993b).

Other proposals for forcing treatment have included making psychiatric patients' welfare benefits contingent upon their compliance with treatment (Thompson, 1996).

It is particularly noteworthy that the use of force to increase compliance has only been proposed in relation to mental health problems. No-one has suggested forcibly medicating or withdrawing the benefits of someone who fails to attend for ante-natal checks or adhere to the diet and insulin regime required by their diabetes. The equally high economic and social costs of 'failure to comply' with treatment and health promotion regimes in physical health areas have never been met with such suggestions. Although there have been isolated incidents when treatment has been denied to people with physical health problems, e.g. to smokers, the subsequent public outcry has deterred large-scale action of this kind. The assumption seems to be that people with physical illnesses can make responsible decisions for themselves whilst those with mental health problems cannot.

Further use of force in relation to psychiatric services is likely to worsen relationships between community services and those whom they serve. If people are forced to take medication by mental health services, then they are likely to withdraw completely from services and avoid contact with them as far as they can. This means that they will fail to receive not only medication but also other types of help. Ideas about, for example, making welfare benefits contingent upon taking medication would not only contravene the civil rights of people with mental health problems, but would clearly worsen the situation of an already disadvantaged group of individuals and increase the general cost to communities. Without money, one cannot pay rent or buy food... so the only options are sleeping rough and begging or stealing to survive.

From a less draconian perspective, a variety of interventions have been used in attempts to increase compliance. For some time it has been assumed that, if people are non-compliant with oral medication (or it is anticipated that they might be) long-acting injections of depot medication should be given instead of pills. It is generally thought that it will be easier to get a person to have an injection once every few weeks than to take pills every day, and at least if the person has an injection the professionals will know that he/she has had it. However, Babiker (1986) has noted the lack of systematic research to justify the routine clinical practice of prescribing depot medication to those who it is thought will not comply with oral medication. Sandford (1996) and Gardner and Hill (1994) demonstrated high rates of non-compliance among outpatients with a diagnosis of schizophrenia who were on depot medication. Further, MacPherson *et al.* (1997) found a trend for patients on depot antipsychotic medication to be more likely to refuse their treatment than those on only oral antipsychotics.

It seems likely that issues of power may be important in relation to depot and oral medication. With depot injections a greater degree of control rests with the mental health professional, while with oral medication more power lies with the person receiving the drug. One of the things that service users most often complain about in relation to psychiatric services is lack of control (Campbell, 1996c). With each dose of oral medication the person has control over whether or not to take it. Such control may, perhaps paradoxically, increase the likelihood that they will take it: they have the choice and they are exercising this choice just as much in taking the pills as in not doing so.

Some 'therapies' have focused on the actual taking of medication (Eckman *et al.*, 1992) and developed behaviourally oriented programmes for people on how to manage drug treatment. Such an approach may be effective for those who wish to take medication but have difficulty in doing so – remembering what to take, when etc., a problem encountered by many people, not only those with mental health problems. However, if a person does not wish to take drugs then no amount of knowing how to manage their drug treatment is likely to make them take them.

Seltzer *et al.* (1980) used a variety of psycho-educational approaches to increase compliance. Such approaches are predicated on the assumption that it must be ignorance on the part of the person that stops them taking medication: if people understand why they should be taking the drugs and the potential consequences of not doing so, then they will take them. While lack of information is a problem often reported by service users (Read and Reynolds, 1996) the assumption that with a full understanding of medication service users will agree with their doctors is not valid. The provision of full information in an accessible and comprehensible form is important – people need to know the pros and cons of taking particular medications in order to make informed choices. However, to confuse informed choice and compliance is a mistake.

Sometimes, psycho-educational approaches consider only a proportion of the information available, for example focusing on the problems of relapse if a person does not take their medication rather than on the problems of permanently living with unpleasant side-effects if they do. Psycho-educational approaches also often focus on one specific model of the problems that they are addressing – usually a neurochemical one – to the exclusion of other available explanations. In such instances the person is not receiving the full information they require to make informed choices: they are being given limited information designed to sway their choices in favour of taking drugs. Psycho-education then becomes simply a form of manipulation and control.

If a psycho-educational approach does ensure that the person has access to full information, then it must be accepted that their informed choice may be in favour of, or against, taking medication. Both are equally valid outcomes. This then ceases to be a means of ensuring compliance but the process of giving people information and helping them to come to a decision that is right for them. Some may decide that, for them, relapses tend to happen when they stop medication and that the negative consequences of these are worse than the negative consequences of the medication. Others may decide that they do not want to permanently take medication or live with its side-effects, but will take it when things start to get worse. Yet others will decide that they wish to live through their good periods and their disturbed ones without drugs and to experience both as important facets of their life.

The choices are, in reality, not limited to taking drugs or not doing so. It is also important to give people choices over which drugs, how much, when and how. Different people experience different side-effects, find different side-effects more or less debilitating and have different preferences about their medication regimes. These should be taken seriously in enabling people to make choices and, of course, everyone has the right to change their mind from time to time. The real decisions are in fact more complex than 'compliance' and 'non-compliance'.

Compliance therapy

There have been recent developments in approaches to improve compliance with prescribed drugs. Kemp *et al.* (1996) reported a cognitive-behavioural 'compliance therapy' based on the type of 'motivational interviewing' that has been used extensively within the drug and substance abuse fields. Rollnick and Miller (1995) define motivational interviewing as *'a directive, client-centred counselling style for eliciting behaviour change by helping clients to explore and resolve ambivalence'*. Such an approach is characterized by a series of principles:

- motivation to change is elicited from the person, not imposed from without
- it is the user's task, not the counsellor's, to articulate and resolve his or her ambivalence
- direct persuasion is not an effective method for resolving ambivalence
- the counselling style is generally a quiet, eliciting one
- the counsellor is directive in helping the person to examine and resolve his or her ambivalence
- readiness to change is not a trait in the user but a fluctuating product of interpersonal interaction
- the therapeutic relationship is more like a partnership or companionship than expert/recipient roles.

However, in moving from the field of substance misuse to trying to make people comply with medication in a psychiatric setting, Kemp *et al.* were forced to considerably compromise the original motivational interviewing model. First, motivational interviewing is predicated on the notion of ambivalence: a conflict between two courses of action such as indulgence and restraint. Although they say that in the third and fourth sessions of their six session intervention *'the benefits and drawbacks of drug treatment were considered and the patient's ambivalence was explored'*, they give no evidence that patients were ambivalent. The large number who were compulsorily detained may suggest that many may have actively decided that they did not want to take medication.

Second, motivational interviewing places great stress on the user, not the counsellor, to articulate and resolve his or her ambivalence and on the therapeutic relationship being one of partnership rather than expert and recipient. The 'modifications' made by Kemp *et al.* to render motivational interviewing relevant to compliance with medication would seem to significantly contravene these premises. They argue that a *'more active problem solving stance'* was adopted with *'guided problem solving'* and an *'increased educational component'*, all more akin to the 'direct persuasion' that Rollnick and Miller counsel against. Further, they report that *'the therapist highlighted discrepancy between patient's actions and beliefs, focusing on adaptive behaviours'*. This is quite contrary to the motivational interviewing premise that it should be the user, not the therapist, who articulates and resolves ambivalence.

Third, there has been debate in the literature on motivational interviewing about the problems and ethical issues which arise if a therapist is intervening towards a different goal than the user and the coercion that this involves (Miller, 1994; Withers, 1995; Miller, 1995). The essence of motivational interviewing is to help people to explore and resolve ambivalence whilst always affirming their freedom, choice and self-direction (Rollnick and Miller, 1995). Significant ethical problems arise where no such ambivalence exists. 'Compliance therapy' has already defined the goal for the user: compliance with medication. The aim cannot, therefore, be to help the person to explore and resolve ambivalence around medication (if they have any) as the acceptable resolution is defined in the nature of the beast: taking medication.

Finally, adding to the ethical problems, we wonder how the therapy was presented? We doubt that there would have been many takers had people been offered 'compliance therapy' yet this is how the intervention was entitled when published (Kemp *et al.*, 1996). Indeed the whole idea of 'compliance therapy' may be at odds with what is generally regarded as therapy. The aim of therapy is to help people to resolve difficulties they have and to reduce distress. Compliance therapy, on the other hand, is designed to make people comply with another form of treatment – medication.

Clearly, it is important to give people the time, space and information to weigh up how they are going to manage and live with their mental distress and disability (Perkins and Repper, 1996). However, informed choice is obviated if the only valid goal of such consideration is compliance with the drug regime prescribed by the doctor. The very idea of 'compliance therapy' wreaks of something that, if practised in a totalitarian state, might be described as brainwashing! Many of the difficulties lie in the very concept of compliance.

The nature of compliance

Haynes *et al.* (1979) defined compliance as:

'the extent to which a person's behaviour... coincides with medical or health advice.'

The assumption is that it is only sensible for people to comply with medical recommendations so that they might avoid, or obtain relief from, illness. It is often tempting for mental health professionals to see 'non-compliance' as something peculiar to people with mental health problems. However, levels of 'non-compliance' in the physical health arena are not dissimilar to those in the mental health field. Podell (1975) calculated that, in relation to physical health prescriptions, an average of only one-third of patients correctly follow physicians' directions. Sackett (1976) in his review of literature in the area showed that, in relation to physical health problems, scheduled appointments are missed 10–50% of the time and about 50% of patients do not take their prescribed medications in accordance with instructions.

Often compliance is discussed in all or nothing terms: either a person does what is prescribed or they do not. This would seem to be a mistake. MacPherson *et al.* (1997) show how a small group of people actively refuse medication while others show a pattern of what has been termed 'partial compliance' taking much, but not all, of that which is prescribed. For example, the authors knew a young man who did not like to take medication regularly but took it when his 'head felt empty'. Often a desire to control on the part of clinicians prevents this type of 'partial compliance': there were those in the team who felt this young man should take his medication 'properly' or not at all. Indeed, when such an approach was followed he received no medication and quickly relapsed, requiring re-admission to hospital. Taking part of his medication may not have minimized his symptoms, but he felt it minimized the side-effects and it did allow him to live outside the hospital: in fact he actually took approximately two-thirds of the medication that was prescribed.

It is further interesting to note that in two studies (Hoge *et al.*, 1990; MacPherson *et al.*, 1997) most of those who refused drugs for a period eventually accepted them voluntarily without the benefits of 'compliance therapy' – people will change their minds and make decisions based on their own experience. Our role is to provide them with full and honest answers to their questions in a manner which they understand so that they can make a choice for themselves, even if that choice is to reject treatment offered.

Some of the factors that have been associated with medication compliance include the complexity of the drug regime (Blackwell, 1972; Eisen and Miller, 1990), the presence of overt side-effects (Blackwell, 1972; Fleischhaker *et al.*, 1994) and more subtle side-effects (Awad, 1993), resistance to the idea of needing medication (Donovan and Blake, 1992), the relationship with the prescriber (Blackwell, 1972; Garrity, 1981; Frank *et al.*, 1995), social support (Blackwell, 1972; Hogarty *et al.*, 1979), more severe social psychopathology (Blackwell, 1972) and the person's more active involvement in medication management (Conrad, 1985).

In clinical practice there is a tendency to see non-compliance with medication as some irrational act resulting from a defect in the individual: their 'personality', 'lack of insight', 'lack of motivation', 'lack of appreciation of the importance of medication'. There is a general assumption that compliance with professionals' advice and prescriptions is the only rational response. Non-compliance becomes pathologized thus requiring a specific aetiology. Indeed Ryan (1986) describes *'four general categories of the aetiology of non-compliance'* including alteration in cognition, alteration in perception, inadequacies in the social system and deficits in the healthcare system. The possibility of non-compliance being a rational response is not considered.

However, several writers have argued that greater attention should be paid to the service user's point of view in issues relating to medication (Janz and Becker, 1984; Leventhal *et al.*, 1992). MacPherson *et al.* (1997) found a strong correlation between compliance, attitudes towards illness and attitudes towards treatment. Ruscher *et al.* (1997) found that the most common reasons given for stopping medication were opposition to the idea of taking medication and a belief that medication did not work, followed by physical side-effects. Further, they found that users' opinions about why other users discontinue their medication most often centred on the idea that the medications did not work. Ruscher *et al.* (1997) argue that this finding supports the view expressed by Diamond (1983) that:

'clinicians may sometimes be too quick to blame non-compliance rather than non-effectiveness when drugs do not help a psychiatric patient.'

A useful framework for understanding people's attitudes and behaviour in relation to mental health problems and treatment may be found in the health belief model developed to understand similar factors in relation to physical health (Becker, 1974). This model starts from the premise that non-compliance is a rational, rather than irrational, act.

Non-compliance as a rational act

To provide a framework of the conditions under which people will or will not follow health recommendations, Kasl and Cobb (1966) distinguished between types of health-related behaviour:

- **preventive behaviour:** activities undertaken by people who believe themselves to be healthy for the purpose of preventing disease or detecting it when they have no symptoms
- **illness behaviour:** activities undertaken by people who feel ill for the purpose of defining what is wrong with them and finding a suitable remedy
- **sick role behaviour:** activities undertaken by those who consider themselves ill for the purposes of getting well.

Preventive behaviour

In most instances, psychiatric literature on compliance relates to people with serious mental health problems taking medication when they are (relatively) 'well' in order to prevent them becoming 'ill', again medication regimes directed towards the maintenance of health rather than the curing of illness. Within the health belief model developed by Becker such decisions are called 'preventive health behaviour' and are influenced by:

- the person's perceived susceptibility to the particular problems: their judgement about how likely it is that they will develop the difficulties
- their judgement about the severity of the consequences of developing the problems
- their evaluation of the feasibility and efficacy of the proposed treatment *versus* their judgement about its costs
- any cues to action that prompt the person to take the treatment.

Within this framework, someone who does not think they will get ill again is unlikely to see the point in continuing to take drugs. This is a quite understandable position. Typically, drugs are seen as curing illness and something to be taken for a short period of time until one is well and then stopped. We know of many people who have taken drugs to resolve acute difficulties but who cannot see the point in continuing to take them when these problems have been resolved. Unfortunately, there are no drugs which cure serious mental health problems (in the same way as antibiotics may cure an infection) but it is all too often the case that this fact has not been communicated to the people who take the drugs. Perhaps it is difficult for clinicians to admit that they are unable to provide cures, but it is certainly necessary if people are to have the information which they need to make judgements about how likely they are to develop problems again and their susceptibility.

Further, in judging susceptibility people need to understand the multi-causal nature of all 'disease', both mental and physical, and the complex interactions of physical, psychological, social and environmental events that are influential in relapse. For example, in relation to mental health problems the emotional environment in which a person lives is important (Leff and Vaughn, 1985), as are the social stressors in their lives (Brown and Birley, 1968; Birchwood et al., 1992; Davey, 1994) and the way in which they deal with these (Birchwood et al., 1988; Birchwood and Shepherd, 1992), the presence of work (Rowland and Perkins, 1988; Grove, 1997) or something to do during the day (Wing and Brown, 1970) and the presence of social supports (Ganster and Victor, 1988). Neurochemicals are one of a variety of factors that may be important in maintaining mental health in someone who experiences serious cognitive and emotional problems.

In relation to decisions about taking maintenance medication, a person's judgements about the severity of the consequences of relapse are probably weighed against the perceived costs and benefits of the proposed treatment. A number of people remain symptomatic despite taking medication, others have learned that they relapse while taking medication. It would be entirely logical for such people to be reluctant to take drugs on a long-term basis especially if, in addition, the medication caused them to feel bad and experience unacceptable side-effects. If, in a person's judgement, the costs of taking the treatment are more than the costs of relapse then it is rational for them not to take the drugs (Pratt, 1998).

Illness behaviour

Whatever the course selected by a person with mental health problems, there may come a time when they need to seek help because their difficulties have worsened. It should be remembered that this can happen even if the person has reliably taken the drugs as prescribed by the doctor.

The timing of decisions to seek help is an important aspect of illness behaviour and can be crucial. Factors like the ease of access to healthcare (Aday and Andersen, 1974), quality of relationship between patient and doctor (Antonovsky and Hartman, 1974) or other clinicians and cultural factors which influence perceptions of health-care offered (Mechanic, 1972) are important in this regard. The extent to which services are accessible and acceptable to those who need them is important if people with serious mental health problems are to receive early help in the event of an exacerbation of their difficulties, whether or not they have chosen to follow the prescriptions of clinicians. Such relationships are likely to be jeopardized by a destructive cycle of force in which the person is compulsorily hospitalized and treated when they cannot be accommodated within their community, leaves hospital as soon as possible and has as little to do with what they perceive as punitive services until once again they are compulsorily detained.

Whether a person is compliant or not, an alternative approach is possible. First, clinicians can work with the person to help them monitor their own problems and know when things are going wrong. Birchwood (1998) has shown that many people are good at monitoring what is happening to them and it is possible for relatives and friends to help as well. Not only does this give an individual the knowledge of when it may be necessary to seek help, but it also allows them to gain a greater understanding and control over their problems. Second, clinicians can work with people to develop 'crisis plans': joint strategies of how they will get help and what will happen if things get bad (Lindow, 1996; Bryant and McClelland, 1997). This too allows a person to be better able to predict and control their crises.

Sick role behaviour

When an illness has been diagnosed and a course of treatment proposed, the individual's perception of the threat posed by the symptoms becomes central (Becker and Rosenstock, 1984). It is in relation to this perceived threat that possible actions and their costs – including following the advice of the clinician – are evaluated and decisions made. In this context, the person's belief in their diagnosis, its implications and the severity of problems seems to be important in relation to a variety of physical health conditions: rheumatic fever (Heinzelman, 1962), asthma (Becker et al., 1978), hypertension (Kirscht and Rosenstock, 1977), renal disease (Hartmann and Becker, 1978). It seems likely that such variables are equally important in relation to serious ongoing mental health problems.

A considerable number of people do not believe themselves to have mental health difficulties of any sort (Taylor and Perkins, 1991) or not the type of problems their diagnosis suggests (Moodley and Perkins, 1991; Perkins and Moodley, 1993). Equally, many do not consider their difficulties to be as severe as their clinicians indicate. Given prevailing social norms, a diagnosis of serious mental health problems – schizophrenia, manic-depressive illness – is often experienced as horrifying to the person to whom it is applied. It is hardly surprising that it will be rejected, along with the implications portrayed in the media, by many who receive it. Such an action is entirely understandable. Further, there is a considerable amount of academic and clinical criticism of such entities as schizophrenia (Bentall *et al.*, 1988; Boyle 1990). Service users are not alone in their rejection of the concept.

Becker and Rosenstock (1984) discuss a persons 'right' to non-compliance and consider some examples of circumstances in which the non-compliant patient is better off. These include *'mis-diagnosis or inappropriate prescribing'* and when *'the patient experiences substantial adverse reactions or side-effects…'*. Although these examples were given in relation to physical health conditions, they would appear to have some relevance in relation to mental health.

Alliance not compliance

Despite the certainty of assertions relating to the necessity for compliance (Kemp *et al.*, 1996), the whole idea is extremely problematic. First, it is predicated on the assumption that the doctor is always right and the patient is wrong, unless they do what the doctor says. In the latter instance, the patient is deemed to have insight, in the former they are considered irrational and lacking in understanding and insight. Such a perspective cannot be squared with concepts such as informed choice: a person having access to the range of information they require in order to make their own decisions about their lives.

The question that ideas about compliance raise is, if the drugs are so good, why should anyone refuse to take them? The reality is that the drugs are not that good. They may suppress the symptoms of some people but they do not cure their difficulties. They also have unpleasant side-effects and may make people feel awful. In such a situation, it is likely that some people will find the symptoms so unpleasant that they will choose to put up with the side-effects to gain some relief. But it is an equally rational decision for a person to decide that the symptom suppressant properties are not worth the side-effects on a long-term basis.

False dichotomies are dangerous. Some people may find one type of drug more tolerable than another and they should be able to try out a range of different prescriptions, dosages, routes, to find the one that suits them. Similarly, some people will be prepared to take drugs when they begin to relapse but not in between times (because of the side-effects). Some people who have taken drugs for a long period of time will want to try stopping them to see if they really need them. Clearly the person could do this themselves but it might be preferable for all concerned if the trial were a collaborative exercise. All these negotiations involve close alliance between the person and their prescriber, working together to sort out what suits the individual.

Finally, drugs are not the only important factor in helping someone to live with their ongoing mental health problems. There are many other ways in which people can be offered help that will decrease the likelihood of relapse: practical help to get decent housing, enough money, assistance with the practicalities of daily life, help to develop social networks and use community facilities, help to find work and education, counselling, therapy and emotional support, somewhere to go and someone to help when things get difficult.

Clearly, any individual faced with living with serious mental health problems has some very hard thinking to do, some difficult decisions to make and perhaps some risky experiments to try. Anyone in such a situation might value an ally who could help them to work through the issues involved and come to decisions that are right for them. Having decided on a course of action, the person may well then require cues to action – assistance that will enable them to carry through their chosen course and help them to review their decisions from time to time in the light of events. But this is not compliance, rather collaborative alliance.

7

Involving service users: influence and incorporation

Despite an increased recognition that there are many stakeholders in the mental health enterprise, 'professionalism' in this, as in other areas of life, remains deep-rooted.

'There is a pervasive societal belief that trained professionals are the only people who know how to provide proper assistance. This attitude exists whether our television needs to be fixed or we need help dealing with personal issues. We have grown accustomed to turning to professionals for help because we assume they have special expertise.' (Besio *et al.*, 1987)

Indeed, such has been the confidence in psychiatric 'experts' that it is often considered impertinent to request that they justify their recommendations: What is the precise likelihood of this intervention having the desired outcome? What is the probability of particular undesired outcomes or side-effects? Too often it is assumed that the 'clinical judgement' of the individual professional – 'in my expert opinion' – should suffice. Yet what is this expertise?

Mental health professionals – whether they be psychiatrists, psychologists, nurses, social workers, counsellors or other therapists – have a very particular form of expertise. They are experts in interpreting the experience of those who use mental health services within the frameworks that their professions have invented (Greenwood, 1957; Ridgeway, 1988; Kitzinger and Perkins, 1993). Psychiatrists, for example, have traditionally developed models of mental distress as brain disease and neurochemical imbalance, so they look for signs and symptoms of such malfunctions and seek to intervene with drugs and physical therapies to put matters right. Psychologists and psychotherapists have invoked a variety of psychological and intrapsychic processes to explain distress, while others adopt more social, familial or interpersonal accounts.

A range of different and often mutually contradictory professional models is available, yet they all share one feature. All were developed by people who had not experienced the phenomena they sought to describe – mental distress and disability – in order to explain the experiences of those who had. A number of people who have had mental health problems are writing about these experiences (Read and Reynolds, 1996) and the gulf between these accounts and the descriptions offered by traditional psychiatry is immense. O'Hagan (1996) offers a unique perspective on this discrepancy when she puts together notes from her own diary with those from her medical file both of which were written during an inpatient admission. For example, she wrote in her diary of the time:

'Today I wanted to die. Everything was hurting. My body was screaming. I saw the doctor. I said nothing. Now I feel terrible. Nothing seems good and nothing good seems possible. I am stuck in a twilight mood where I go down like the setting sun into a lonely black hole where there is room for only one.'

At the same time her hospital file reported:

'Flat, lacking in motivation, sleep and appetite good. Discussed aetiology. Cont. LiCarb. 250 mg qid. Levels next time.' (O'Hagan, 1996)

Increasingly, those who experience mental health problems are questioning the wisdom of professional judgements and many are turning to alternative sources of expertise: others who have experienced mental distress and disability (Chamberlin, 1977, 1990).

'Ex-patients… are beginning to turn to each other rather than to mental health professionals for emotional and instrumental support. They are finding that often people with experiential knowledge (i.e. having learned through personal experience) are more able to understand their needs than are professionals who have learned through education and training. Moreover, they are finding the support and help they give each other to be as valuable – or sometimes more valuable – than the interventions of trained professionals.' (Besio et al., 1987)

Such moves can be seen in a variety of self-help and user-run services (Lindow, 1994) and organizations such as Survivors Speak Out, the UK Advocacy Network, MINDLINK, the National Self-Harm Network and the Hearing Voices Network.

The role of users in mental health services

Traditionally, people who experience mental distress and disability have only been the recipients of treatments administered by the professionals who run mental health services. However, the growth of the user/survivor movement has enabled many to speak out about the shortcomings of such services and resulted in demands for a greater say in what happens: for choice, control and power to determine the type and style of treatment, support and services offered. Unfortunately, given prevailing societal attitudes towards people who experience mental health problems (Read, 1996) a user voice, where it exists, has been hard won. There are many within services who continue to disregard the expertise of personal experience, especially where it runs counter to deeply held tenets of their profession or practice.

Some services apparently see the involvement of users as an act of altruism – 'It is good and kind for fortunate professionals to ask their less fortunate users what they feel, think or want.' User involvement is not seen as the right of people who use services nor as essential to the running of an effective service but as a mark of good practice and something to be over-ruled if users, in the eyes of professionals, are mistaken. As Edna Conlan (1996) describes:

'There are times when, as someone who has been and still is a recipient of mental health services trying to work with mental health services to empower service users, I feel as though I am shaking hands with the devil. The feeling tends to be strongest when I find myself sitting on a high-powered committee which is intent on sending out signals that the mere presence of people using the services is evidence of its goodwill and obvious commitment to delivering user-centred services.'

Alternatively, user involvement may be construed by services as an 'optional extra'. Within such a perspective resources may only be allocated to involving users if everything else is adequately funded. There are few services where it can be demonstrated that a clinical post, for example, has been cut in order to provide funds for a Patients' Council or advocacy worker, or where a professional-run service has been cut to enable a user-led service to be funded. In an era when resources for mental health are unlikely to increase, if user involvement and user-run services are to become a reality then it will be necessary to *stop* doing some things in order to release resources to *start* doing others.

In most services, pressures exist to be seen to be doing something about user involvement but too often this does not involve any real commitment to establishing the structures and organization to enable such involvement to become a reality. Token individuals may be invited onto committees, or groups of users 'rounded up' for particular planning events. However, without proper ongoing fora – organizations and networks through which the diverse views of the user/survivor constituency can be tapped – the position of these token representatives is considerably weakened.

The number of people who complain about their experience of mental health services, together with the number who use them only when compelled to do so or who avoid them as far as possible, cannot be ignored. If services are to remain relevant to those who experience mental distress and disability, the involvement of these people is necessary to their survival: not as an act of altruism or the icing on the cake, but as an essential ingredient of the cake itself. User involvement cannot be an act of token window dressing, but must be a process of establishing structures to tap and attend to user expertise and really ensure that it can and does shape the services offered.

Many important gains have been won through the efforts of users and survivors:

'The growth of the user movement and the active campaigning, advocacy and development work of local and national groups, has ensured that users are now considered legitimate participants in planning, consultation and service delivery, at least in some areas.' (Beeforth, Conlan and Graley, 1994)

Indeed, Campbell (1997) suggests that user involvement in the late 1990s is extensive:

'The voices of significant numbers of users can be heard through the hundreds of local user-led action groups... The Disabled Persons Act 1986 and the NHS and Community Care Act have made consultation a necessity. Mental health service users have been involved in the Mental Health Nursing Review and the Mental Health Task Force and in giving evidence to the DoH and parliamentary reviews of mental health legislation.'

However, presence does not necessarily equate with influence. Campbell (1997) goes on to say that:

'... deciding the quality, as opposed to the quantity, of involvement is more difficult.'

Despite good intentions and sterling efforts, the power relations that exist within services remain fundamentally unchanged. So, for example, while a user may be consulted on their views about treatment, they do not have any right to insist that their views are incorporated into the care that they receive.

'I can talk, but I may not be heard. I can make suggestions, but they may not be taken seriously. I can voice my thoughts, but they may be seen as delusions. I can recite my experiences, but they may be interpreted as fantasies. To be a patient or even an ex-client is to be discounted.' (Leete, 1988)

The fundamental dilemma for clinicians in involving service users in the design and running of mental health services rests once again on the notion of power. It is impossible for users to gain more influence in determining what is offered without professionals and managers losing some of their power, and giving up power can be hard.

Changing the balance of power

Changes in power relationships between users and providers are of the essence. Although these can be difficult to achieve, there is a great deal that can be done and three areas seem to be important: information, influencing and changing existing services, and establishing alternative services.

Information

Information brings power and one of the most common complaints from service users revolves around lack of information (Rogers *et al.*, 1993; Read, 1996). Most of all, users want information on the effects and side-effects of medication, alternatives to medication, the range of services available and rights, especially those to receive or refuse treatment (Read, 1996).

While the provision of information seems basic, most people working within and using mental health services agree that it is often in short supply. There are several dilemmas associated with the provision of information. First, there is the 'problem' that if people are given information about treatments and services they may wish to use them! This not only challenges professionals' right to decide who gets what, but also challenges providers' ability to supply what is demanded. There are often shortages and some therapies and services may not be available at all. This raises questions about whether it is appropriate to inform people about things that they cannot have. On the one hand, it could be argued that this simply leads to disappointment and unnecessary distress. On the other hand, it could be argued that people have a right to know about the range of options that may be helpful so that, if these are not available locally, they have the information they need to campaign to make them available.

Second, there are issues about how and when to give people information in a form that will be comprehensible to them. For example, to be told of one's diagnosis and treatment options in a large case conference under the gaze of a dozen or so clinicians is hardly conducive to the processing of any information given. If a person is distressed or disabled, the process of making choices about what they want may be a protracted one requiring time on the part of clinicians or other helpers. It may be considered easier all round if the information they are given is weighted in some way to help them make a decision, or only part of the information is given. However, whenever partial or incomplete information is offered, the individual is deprived of choice and agency. If someone is in an acute crisis they may be temporarily unable to process the information they need to make the necessary decisions. In such circumstances, they may nominate a friend or family member who can be involved in making decisions with them.

Third, and most especially, information is not a value-free commodity. The 'facts' depend upon the position, knowledge, attitude and views of the person recounting them, therefore the issues of who provides information, when, to whom and how are important. For example, some information is produced by the drug companies trying to sell their wares and is therefore unlikely to offer an unbiased account. However, such problems are not limited to medication. Descriptions of services, facilities and treatments, including talking treatments, are typically written by providers of these who are likely to have both an economic and a professional stake in what they are doing and present it in a favourable light.

When purchasing goods and services most people would prefer to look further than the manufacturer or retailer's 'blurb'. They might consult a less biased source, e.g. a consumer magazine, or people who already use the goods or services. The same might usefully apply when considering different treatments and services. For example, the *Patient Factsheet* on electro-convulsive therapy (ECT) produced by the Royal College of Psychiatrists (1993a) and supported by an educational grant from the drug company Lundbeck Limited, describes ECT as *'the most effective treatment for severe depression'* and, after describing some short-term effects such as recent memory problems and confusion, it says *'ECT does not have any long-term effects on your memory or intelligence'.* While this would accord with the experience of one of the current authors (Perkins, 1994), it is not consistent with that of others. For example, GM (1994) said:

'No-one knew why it worked but it did, they said. It would do me good they said. What they did not say was this: 1 Waking up with a head full of wet cement. 2 My jaw feeling like I had chewed half a hundredweight of Beech, not chewing gum. 3 Forgetting things that had happened. 4 Remembering things that had happened.'

Taylor (1996) also describes distressing short-term confusion and memory loss, together with lasting difficulties of a type completely denied in the Royal College of Psychiatrists' leaflet:

'Even to this day I may be in the middle of a conversation when I forget what I am talking about and have to put much effort into remembering, or be reminded by my best friend. Often I enter a room and forget what I am doing there. I am convinced that ECT played a large part in the problems which I have experienced...'

He goes on to make it clear that, in writing of his experiences:

'It is not my wish to hurt or offend people who have had ECT and who have obtained short-term benefits. However, I am stating that whilst ECT seems to work in some cases, it certainly did not work for myself or others like me. Therefore, for any person to state that it is safe, reliable and effective for all people is a travesty of the truth.'

The same might apply to any other intervention or service. Some people derive great benefit from drugs, others experience alarming side-effects. While it is assumed that 'talking treatments' are relatively benign in terms of undesired side-effects, this is not a universally held perspective (Masson, 1988; Kitzinger and Perkins, 1993) and there exist numerous accounts of abuse by therapists of their clients. For example, studies show that 15% of therapists admit to sexual contact with a client – how many do not admit it? (Bouhoustos *et al.*, 1983). Such information is rarely listed as an 'undesired side-effect' of psychotherapy.

Full information is important in relation to all supports, services and sources of help within the mental health arena. Information should include:

- evidence of effectiveness – the likelihood of a person achieving different goals via its use
- potential detrimental (side) effects
- alternative strategies and approaches that might be adopted
- what the experience of the treatment is like.

For example, having a CPN visit may provide support and someone to talk to, but there is little evidence that this has beneficial effects on symptoms or functioning (Brooker *et al.*, 1996). Further, having a mental health professional visit might be stigmatizing if, for example, neighbours see them and it might reinforce the person's feelings of inadequacy. Other ways of obtaining help and support include self-help groups, the Samaritans, friends and ordinary community social, educational and work resources.

In giving information there will often be areas of ignorance and uncertainty. This raises questions about whether the limits of knowledge about a particular intervention should be conveyed. It might be argued that a professional must appear confident in order to encourage service users and give interventions the best chance of success. But this essentially involves lying by omission. It also speaks volumes about the professional's attitude to the user, implying that while the professional can be trusted to weigh evidence, and lack of evidence, and reach a sensible conclusion, the user cannot be relied upon to do so.

Sometimes, in the presence of all the information, a person may defer judgement to someone else about what to do: ask their friend, relative, doctor or nurse what they should do. Increasingly, service users are trusting others who have experienced similar difficulties and the range of information produced by self-help and user groups is rising (MIND, 1986; Frederick, 1991; Manic Depressive Fellowship, 1995; Baker, 1995; Leader, 1995). This means that clinicians can now make available to service users information from a variety of sources.

Finally, it is important to retain a distinction between the giving of information and choice or consultation, both at an individual and a service level. Consultation involves the possibility of influencing outcome, the giving of information does not. If information-giving masquerades as consultation then those involved are immediately devalued as it is known *a priori* that their views will not be heeded. If no choice is being given this should be made clear: at least honesty allows the possibility of protest whereas the illusion of consultation does not.

Influencing and changing existing services

Although the opportunities for 'user participation' have increased since the mid-1980s (Barker and Peck, 1996; Campbell, 1996b; Read, 1996), many users continue to express doubts about the willingness of mental health services to give users decision-making powers (Campbell, 1997). Such concerns seem justified in the light of a review of mental health service user involvement which found little evidence of power sharing within social services (Bowl, 1996). Perkins and Fisher's (1996) audit of care plans provides further support for users' doubts in relation to care plans. In this context independent advocacy can augment the service user's voice.

ADVOCACY

Advocacy is the process through which individuals and groups express their own rights and concerns (Sang and O'Brien, 1984). Three types of advocacy have been described (Bingley, 1990):

- self-advocacy where people assert their own rights either individually or collectively
- citizen advocacy where a lay volunteer represents the needs and interests of someone as if they were their own
- professional advocacy where lawyers or other trained professionals assist people in defending their rights.

To this list might usefully be added peer advocacy where someone who has experienced similar problems to the person concerned represents their interests. It is the notion of peer advocacy which has been developed by The United Kingdom Advocacy Network (UKAN). This user-run network provides training, advice and support in group advocacy through the development of user-run patient councils and support groups, and individual – independent – peer advocacy (Conlan *et al.*, 1994).

Advocacy may be informal, formal (e.g. through administrative complaints procedures, tribunals etc.) or public (influencing national and local policies and service developments through conferences, lobbying and so forth). However, people using services generally adopt a form of informal self-advocacy to request support that they want in a manner which they can use. This approach is markedly limited by the very uneven power relationships that exist between providers and users. It is often difficult for service users to engage in significant disagreements with those who are providing their care – and win. Although this may be due to legal restrictions, it is more often the case that professionals believe that they know best.

If a person is unable to make decisions for his/herself, then it is not uncommon for professionals to consult relatives. No matter how deserving of attention these people might be, they have interests of their own which are distinct from those of the user. It is important to know whether the individual would wish them to speak on their behalf. Although it may be the case that lay volunteers have a certain independence, they too are not without their own views on mental health. The vested interests and biases that these can introduce into the advocacy situation cannot be ignored.

WHAT USERS WANT FROM MENTAL HEALTH SERVICES

If each person is to get the help they want, it is important that a range of supports and services exist. There have been numerous accounts of what users want from services (Rogers *et al.*, 1993; Tanzman, 1993; Campbell, 1996c). Read (1996) draws on these accounts to describe the eight things that service users most want from mental health services.

1 **Information**.
2 **Choice.** Everyone is different: *'Someone who can't sleep may benefit from yoga, sleeping pills, meditation or counselling, but which of those do mental health workers offer?... Above all, time and time again, people say that the choice that is missing is someone to talk to.'*
3 **Accessibility**. People want services near their homes and services that are open when they need them, not simply office hours, Monday to Friday: *'For us, Christmas can be the loneliest time.'*
4 **Advocacy**. People want access to independent advocacy services to put their views across: *'Generally service users are scared of mental health workers. Professionals might not feel very intimidating, but there's something about the relationship we have with you, especially if you're a doctor, which means that we are scared of you.'*
5 **Equal opportunities**. No-one has a monopoly on the truth about mental health, and those who experience mental distress want access to people who will understand their experiences: race, gender, lesbian/gay, class, and age are important. Services need to offer privacy, security and freedom from harassment by staff and other users. Initiatives where service users have been employed as part of clinical teams are also important in this regard (Perkins *et al.*, 1997; Bond *et al.*, 1997).
6 **Income and employment**. Housing and employment schemes that give people money to spend or training and support to get jobs are vital.
7 **Self-help**. Service users need opportunities to support and learn from each other and develop new solutions together (Baker, 1995).
8 **Self-organization**. Service users have a lot to contribute to the design and running of services, and without proper user organizations at local and national level these talents cannot be tapped.

It might be argued that, for as long as most people who experience mental health problems use the mainstream mental health system, it is important that they have a say in how this operates at both an individual and a service level (Perkins, 1996b). However, as users become incorporated into mainstream provision, as they participate in planning, development and care structures whose nature is determined by those services, their radical independent voice is diminished and their impact is weakened.

'There is a danger that this incorporation of the user view into statutory agendas serves to dampen the impact of the user agenda. There is a very real danger that statutory partners will

involve users in the process, *as they are being encouraged to do, but will carefully control, and if necessary dilute the* outcomes *of that dialogue.'* (Barker and Peck, 1996).

It is rare, for example, that users form a majority on any significant planning body, indeed they are more typically in a small minority. This means that they cannot over-rule the decision of the majority of non-users of the group and must make compromises in order to get their voices heard. However, because of their presence in the planning process, the outcomes of that process are leant a 'user involvement' credibility despite the fact that, unless users and other interested parties happen to agree, they do not represent the views of the users involved. An independent critical user/survivor voice is as necessary as user participation in services.

While user participation in the design and running of services has undoubtedly resulted in some gains, Campbell (1996b) argues that any assessment of the success of the user/survivor movement must be conducted within a broader context. He argues that while the credibility and respectability of users in services has increased, there has been little increase in choice in the use of services and control over the physical treatments received. In considering the predicament of users and ex-users outside mental health services – as citizens in the community – he sees the situation in even less optimistic terms:

'The optimism that some of us felt that the public might gain access to and respect for the alternative understandings of people with direct experience of psychosis, eating distress, phobias, self-harm and so on has been largely offset by the work of certain organisations to re-emphasise the supposed alienness of people with such problems... I do not think this is a particularly good time to be "mentally ill" and a citizen of the United Kingdom. (When has it ever been?) What worries me most is that we now seem to be struggling as much to prevent things getting worse as we are to make them better.'

Establishing alternative supports and services

While user efforts to change existing services have generally been most widely discussed, this is probably because they pose relatively little threat to the mental health establishment. Barker and Peck (1996) describe four goals that can be discerned within the user movement. The first two involve engagement with existing services: fighting them (via, for example, campaigning) or fixing them (via, for example, patient councils). These two goals, they argue, have been met to a far greater degree than the latter two: escaping them (via, for example, creating safe houses) and replacing them (with user-led and user-run alternatives). These latter two have barely been addressed, possibly because they involve a very real shift in the balance of power between providers and users/survivors.

User-run and user-controlled alternatives to mainstream provision have a longer history in other countries than they do in the UK (O'Hagan, 1991; Perkins, 1993;

Lindow, 1994). In the Netherlands, the USA, Japan, Canada and New Zealand there are many examples of self-help alternatives that have not only stood the test of time but prospered, sometimes in situations of limited resources that would have caused the demise of most mainstream services (Perkins, 1993). These initiatives span a wide range of areas from support in independent accommodation and residential services through daytime support and employment and vocational training schemes, arts and other creative projects, to schemes to reach homeless people.

Nevertheless, there is reluctance among mainstream purchasers to invest in user-run alternatives. This reflects, at least in part, the threat which such alternatives pose to existing power relations. If users can run their own services, then professionals lose some of their traditional power. However, as Perkins (1996b) has pointed out:

'Changes in power relationships do not mean that professionals have no skills, rather that these skills might be used in a different way... There is a need to move away from the idea of professionals as experts who know best, controlling services and telling patients what to do. An alternative model where professionals place their expertise and services at the disposal of those who need them, is both possible and desirable. This is the model within which many professionals (like lawyers) work.'

In some user-controlled and user-run services (Perkins, 1993) professionals have been employed by the users who run them: a shift from professionals telling users what to do, to users telling professionals what they want. This involves according users expertise and taking seriously what they say. Unfortunately, whether in relation to providing full and frank information, seeking genuine user influence on the shape of existing services or transferring resources to establish user-led alternatives, it is all too common for users to have their views ignored.

Disregarding users/survivors

Ridgeway (1988) argues that the reason why users' perspectives are often ignored in mental health services lies at the level of basic attitudes and social structures. There is the general presumption that incompetence in all spheres of life inevitably accompanies the label of mental illness (Goffman, 1961; Chamberlin, 1977; Leete, 1988). Therefore mental health services have seen their role as acting as some kind of 'benevolent parent' and 'surrogate decision-maker' for those who experience mental distress and disability. This 'provider knows best' perspective is reinforced by professionalism: the belief that the professional has access to a specialized body of knowledge and theory that is not accessible to, and cannot be understood by, non-professionals (Greenwood, 1957).

'When professionals are faced with demands for assistance they feel inadequate to meet, or when their viewpoint or service offerings are rejected, they blame the person's "lack of insight",

"poor motivation", or other character flaws, rather than seeing it as their own inability to understand or respond to their client's life experience. This "blaming the victim" mentality is common across special-needs groups.' (Ridgeway, 1988)

At a day-to-day level there are numerous ways in which the views of users are disregarded by those who provide services. First, those service users who do speak out may be devalued and disregarded because it is asserted that they do not represent all service users. Instead of engaging with the arguments presented, the person, irrespective of what they say, is simply dismissed as unrepresentative:

'"But you're not like my clients." If I had a crisp tenner every time that "argument" was used to counter my entire presentation on increasing the participation of people who use mental health services in the planning and provision of services, I would probably be better paid than those who level the charge… why is so much valuable time and energy wasted on what is little more than a personal attack, the first defence of a frightened traditionalist who hasn't bothered to listen to a word of the twenty-minute presentation that invariably precedes the charges?' (Crepaz-Keay, 1996)

A rich diversity of politics, views, interests and experiences exist among those who experience mental distress, just as it exists among service providers and the population as a whole. No spokesperson from the Royal Colleges of Psychiatrists or Nursing represents their entire profession or even a known proportion of it, yet their views are still seen as worthy of attention. In all organizations, some people, e.g. people from minority racial and ethnic groups, lesbians, gays, and women, find it less easy to get their views heard and attention must be paid to ensuring them a voice. Unanimity among any sizeable group is rare. The existence of disparate views is often seen as a problem – 'We don't know who to believe' – while it might better be seen as a strength: the presence of a richer pool of wisdom and opinions. The more participation by people who experience mental distress and disability is facilitated, resourced and taken seriously, the greater the range of views that will be tapped, and the more extensive the information and ideas available.

Second, there are always arguments about resource constraints. However, it is important to note that many of the things that users/survivors request do not cost money. For example, Campbell (1996c) outlines four themes that emerge when service users talk about crisis services, three of which would cost very little, if anything:

'People want more control, particularly more of their own control, over crisis situations… People want to gain an understanding of and from their crises… People want to be treated with respect and dignity.'

Where there are significant cost implications of what user/survivors want – as in the fourth demand by Campbell for 24-hour non-medical crisis services – decisions have to be made about priorities. In times of plenty it is possible to meet diverse demands simply by adding to the range of services and interventions available. However, resources in mental health services are scarce and it is rarely possible simply to add new services to those which already exist. Hard decisions must be made about whose views take precedence. If users' views are heeded only when there is surplus resource then they will never have a significant say in the shape of services.

Third, there are a variety of arguments used to discredit and devalue users' opinions which are predicated on the notion that the views they espouse are a consequence or symptom of their illness. Dismissing what people say as an indication of their supposed psychopathology is at the very root of most mental health theorizing. Professional models, whether they be medical, nursing, psychological, psychotherapeutic or systemic, typically interpret what users/survivors say in terms of their model or theory about what is wrong with them. On the basis of these interpretations they decide what the person *really* means and therefore needs. This process is bolstered by the concept of 'insight' (Lewis, 1934; David, 1990). As Campbell (1996a) has described:

'The concept of insight – perhaps lack of insight would be most appropriate from the psychiatric perspective – is one of the most powerful and insidious forces eroding our position as competent, creative individuals.'

A person is deemed to have insight if they agree with the professional about the existence, nature and treatment of the malaise. If they do not, then they lack insight and their views can legitimately be disregarded (on treatment and other matters) as simply a manifestation of their 'illness' (Perkins and Moodley, 1993). It is not surprising that 'lack if insight' is frequently used as a justification for compulsory detention and treatment.

It can be argued that there may be brief periods of crisis, profound distress or desperate despair when a person's views and opinions may change and when they construe the world differently. At times their world may diverge from the consensus reality. But it is a shift of unwarranted dimensions to move from this to a position which argues that they have no valid opinions about their experiences and the help that would be appropriate, that they cannot achieve control over their lives and that they are unable to contribute to the design of services in a valid way.

Listening seriously to service users even when their views do not accord with those of professionals is a major challenge facing mental health services. Unfortunately, changing the balance of power within mental health services is made more difficult by the contradictory demands upon those services and their clinicians. The demands that the public be protected from 'dangerous lunatics' and that 'compliance' with treatment is assured do not sit easily with allowing those same service users/survivors to determine the type of help they want and need. However, even without such contradictions, shifting power relationships will pose many dilemmas for professionals who, while they may often feel powerless, are nevertheless used to having the power to determine what they think is right for 'their patients'.

It will always be difficult for a professional to do something that they consider less than optimal, or fail to do something that they believe would be genuinely helpful. It is tempting to seek reasons why the views of those users whose opinions more fundamentally challenge accepted wisdom should be disregarded. However, when a professional regards his or her opinions as superior to those of users, for whatever reason, this by definition prevents the real inclusion of the expertise of personal experience.

8

Health needs, therapy, social care and the practicalities of life

Any service, team or individual clinician must make decisions about how they can best assist each person in their care. In theory, an assessment is performed and on the basis of this priorities are decided and a care plan constructed. However, in reality, the situation is more complex and this complexity presents many dilemmas.

At a very basic level, there is worrying experimental evidence which shows that clinicians may not necessarily base their decisions about what care to provide on information from the assessments they perform (Conning and Rowland, 1992). Instead, decisions about care may be related to the attitudes and beliefs of clinicians. Such experimental findings are supported by data from clinical services (Perkins and Fisher, 1996). Even where clinicians do base their interventions on the assessments they undertake, these assessments do not constitute some value-free 'objective fact'. The assessments performed, the way in which the results are interpreted, and therefore the areas targeted for intervention and support, critically depend on the model or framework that the clinician employs. The intervention and support offered will vary depending on what is assessed, with whom, and how it is interpreted to guide intervention.

Different approaches: different interventions

Different clinicians adopt different models. If, for example, a largely organic framework is adopted, then symptoms will be assessed, the diagnosis determined and the appropriate pharmacological intervention prescribed. Even if other aspects of the person's life are seen as important, it will be assumed that the best way of altering these is by changing the underlying organic pathology. Such a model may be elaborated to consider how the person's 'compliance' with medication can be enhanced (Kemp *et al.*, 1996). The clinician's understanding of symptomatology may also influence intervention, and this may be influenced by the sources of information used: users, their relatives and other staff often give different accounts depending upon their experience and perspective. Even a single framework – one of organic psychiatry – does not automatically lead to the same intervention when employed by different clinicians with their different beliefs and perspectives. It is known that different psychiatrists make different diagnoses when faced with ostensibly the same information (Bentall, 1990).

Such 'cure' perspectives, directed towards the identification and removal of 'symptoms', are not restricted to organic psychiatry: they are equally prevalent in psychological, psychotherapeutic, systemic and counselling approaches. Whatever their construction of the underlying processes involved – neurochemical, psychological, interpersonal – cure-based models are of limited use in working with those who have ongoing mental health problems. Such people have experienced numerous attempts at cure and their difficulties remain. Continual searching for cure can be very dispiriting for staff and user alike and can devalue the person by implying that the only way they can lead a valuable, fulfilling life is if their problems are removed (Ekdawi and Conning, 1994).

Ekdawi and Conning (1994) and Perkins and Repper (1996) outline other models used to guide work with those who experience ongoing mental health problems. In many quarters a 'skills' approach has been popular. Within this perspective the goal is to:

'Provide the disabled person with the physical, intellectual and emotional skills needed to live, learn and work in the community with the least possible amount of support from agents of the helping professions.' (Anthony, 1977)

In this type of model, it is not symptoms which form the basis of assessment but skills: what a person can and cannot do. The skills deficits which prevent the person from functioning effectively are identified, present and required levels of functioning are determined, and then the discrepancy between these is eliminated. The skill is broken down into small steps and then taught in a systematic manner. Instead of a care plan focusing on drugs or measures to enhance compliance or psychological interventions to modify auditory hallucinations and delusional beliefs, a skills approach is based on systematic skills training and practice.

Once again, there are problems with this approach (Ekdawi and Conning, 1994; Perkins and Repper, 1996). For example, it tends to lead to a focus on basic mechanical areas where there are identifiable skills to teach. It generally ignores the cognitive component of skilled performance – deciding what to do, when, how much, getting feedback from performance and adjusting behaviour accordingly, all of which can be profoundly affected in people who have serious and fluctuating cognitive difficulties. Skills training can also tend to infantilize people and there remain problems when an individual fails to learn to perform the skill independently.

The aim of 'maximizing independence' is often adopted in services as if it were some intrinsic good. It is undoubtedly the case that many service users wish to have more control over their lives (Read and Reynolds, 1996) and minimize contact with mental health services to reduce the stigma attached to them (Rose, 1996). But perhaps the aim of maximizing independence from helping professions is misplaced. The wish of service users to minimize contact may say more about the nature of services than the needing of help *per se*.

There are many ways in which people can get help in society that do not reflect negatively on the person who is assisted; indeed some actively enhance their status. Has anyone been demeaned by having a nanny, or a cleaner, or a builder to do the roof, or a pizza delivered, or going out for a meal, or using a service wash? It is perhaps noteworthy that with all of these acceptable forms of help, the user has a considerable degree of control: choice over what to get, when to get it and so forth. The critical question is not whether a person needs help but the quality and value attached to that help and whether it enables them to lead the life they wish to lead.

Problems and needs

Both cure and skills approaches are essentially problem-based: their starting point is that which has gone *wrong* or what the person *cannot* do. Such problem-based approaches to assessment and care planning can be very negative. They prevent clinicians, and often the dispirited service user, from seeing the assets, skills and interests that they have: any positive features are likely to get lost (both literally and figuratively) in a sea of difficulties. If a person is unable to use their skills and pursue their interests then they are at grave risk of losing them (Goffman, 1961; Wing and Brown, 1970). An approach that enables them to do things they want to do, and those which they are good at, is important.

Rapp and his colleagues (Rapp and Wintersteen, 1989) developed a successful model of strengths-based care planning which is structured around what the person wants to achieve and the skills and assets that they have in order to do so. Instead of a plan based on the elimination or minimization of problems, assessment revolves around what the person wants to do ('I want to be a nurse'), where they are now (no formal qualifications), what skills they have (basic literacy and numeracy, enjoys reading, regular contact with sister's children and sometimes looks after them, always dresses well...), and what resources exist in the community that represent opportunities (chance to meet nurses to talk about what training is involved, opportunities for voluntary work at a local luncheon club…). The care plan then involves putting these resources together (or maybe finding others) to help the person move in the direction of their ambitions.

The shift from problem-oriented perspectives towards more positive approaches to assessment and care planning with people who experience serious mental health problems is reflected in the literature. There is now very little mention of 'problems'. Instead the term 'needs' is almost universally favoured (DoH, 1995a; Sainsbury Centre for Mental Health, 1997). This is based on the idea that the extent of a person's unmet needs is assessed and a care plan organized to meet those needs. This approach allows the complex requirements of each individual to be addressed, and once needs have been identified a range of different methods of meeting them might be employed. The destructive failure inherent in cure-based approaches is avoided and there is no necessary value attached to maximizing a person's independence from services.

However, despite the prevalence of 'needs' rhetoric there is no real agreement about what a 'need' is. At one level, lists of 'needs' look like a semantic sleight of hand, problems expressed in a different form: needs to cook instead of can't cook; needs to stop hitting people instead of hits people; needs to go out instead of can't go out. In more extreme form, one recent text (Sainsbury Centre for Mental Health, 1997) listed self-neglect, social withdrawal, slowness, over-activity and challenging behaviour in a chapter entitled *The needs to which services must respond*. If the term 'need' is simply seen as a polite word for 'problem' then a needs approach to assessment and care planning remains problem-based.

Because of the difficulties in defining need, there is a temptation for clinicians to think about needs in terms of service inputs, and when looking at community provision or in social care assessments this is the approach frequently adopted (Brewin *et al.*, 1987, 1988). So people are deemed to need high and low support hostels, nursing homes and so forth. A new breed of human being is born: one who quite unlike any other member of the species has a need for day centres and group homes. The problem here is that a person's needs and the possible means of meeting those needs have become confused. Human needs are many and varied: from personal safety and basic physiological needs, through belonging and companionship, to self-esteem and contentment (Maslow, 1970). Group homes, hostels and day centres are just one way of meeting some of these needs, but there are many others and the alternatives may be preferable.

If the assessment of needs is confused with their solutions then this impedes the provision of individualized support tailored to each person's unique set of requirements. For example, people may 'need' a day centre for a variety of reasons: to provide specific therapeutic inputs, purposeful activity and a structure to their day, company and social contact or somewhere to get a main meal. Each of these can be provided in different settings which for some people may be preferable. Various forms of therapeutic input may be available in GP surgeries or outpatient clinics.

Purposeful activity may better be provided via supported employment (Bond *et al.*, 1997), voluntary work or education. A main meal could just as well be provided at a local café. Social contact can be provided at numerous social clubs and community centres depending on the person's preferences. For example, women often prefer at least some women-only facilities (Perkins *et al.*, 1996; Repper *et al.*, 1997); older people may prefer to be with people of their own age group (irrespective of whether they have mental health problems) and luncheon clubs provide an opportunity for this; and a variety of clubs and organizations provide more appropriate social contact for those from minority ethnic and racial groups.

On the residential side, people may be deemed to 'need' a hostel for many reasons. In particular, they may require *supervision* without which they may be a danger to themselves (for example, poor concentration may lead to such things as leaving the gas on or lighted cigarettes burning). Alternatively, they may have difficulty in organizing the practicalities of everyday life – cooking, cleaning, food and so forth – and require *support* in doing these things. Yet again, they may also seek company and social contact. If a person requires continual supervision then it may be the case that someone has to be around all the time in their accommodation. However, if it is support or company they need then this may not be the case. It is entirely possible to help someone organize the basics of daily living by support in their own home – and this is the thing that most people, quite naturally, want (Meltzer *et al.*, 1991; Beeforth *et al.*, 1990). Similarly, if someone needs company then they could be helped to go out and get this (most of us do not live with our friends) or could live in a non-staffed shared flat or house.

All shared psychiatric facilities, whether they be in the community or not, constitute, to a greater or lesser extent, 'block treatment': they provide a single facility for people with a range of different needs that could be met elsewhere and by other means. A day centre or a hostel may be the best way of meeting a particular person's needs but it may not. Unfortunately, alternative possibilities are not considered if needs are hidden in terms of their solutions and the person is deemed to require a particular facility.

A further problem with the concept of need revolves around what constitutes a 'need' and what constitutes a 'want' or a 'wish'? While most people could probably agree on basic physiological needs, issues become somewhat murky beyond this point. Is a home of one's own a basic need? What about needs for work? And personal safety? Hospitals and psychiatric facilities can be very dangerous places (Wood and Copperman, 1996; Nibert *et al.*, 1989). What sort of an income is a basic necessity? In many community residential facilities the basic income of around £13 per week does not allow people to smoke, go out and use facilities in the community or clothe themselves decently – but maybe these are not basic needs? In times of great pressure on mental health and social services budgets, judgements about need necessarily become coloured by the amount of money available. So needs assessments become, at least in part, an economic assessment.

Social disability and access

A further model originating from the work of Wing and colleagues (1962, 1978, 1981) and developed by Perkins and Dilks (1992) and, more recently, by Perkins and Repper (1996), rests on the construct of disability and has strong parallels with frameworks used in the field of physical disability. A person who experiences physical limitations is physically disabled in so far as they are unable to negotiate the demands of the ordinary (able-bodied) physical world without help, support and adaptation of that world. Someone who experiences the cognitive and emotional problems associated with ongoing mental health difficulties is socially disabled in so far as they are unable to negotiate the demands and expectations of the ordinary (able-minded) social world without help, support and adaptation of that world. Whether a person is physically or socially disabled, the purpose of treatment, intervention and support is to ensure that the individual has access to those opportunities they desire and is able to develop, grow and make best use of their skills and abilities.

It should be noted that in both the 1992 Americans with Disabilities Act and the 1995 UK Disability Discrimination Act, 'psychiatric' disability is included alongside physical disability and there is a requirement for organizations to make 'reasonable accommodations' (USA) or 'reasonable adjustments' (UK) to ensure that disabled people have access. There has been substantial consideration of what access might mean for someone who experiences physical disabilities, but this has not been the case for those who are socially disabled by ongoing mental health problems. Access to the social world involves access to those social facilities, roles, relationships and activities that are relevant for the individual.

Within such a model, assessment is a four-stage process:

1 Identification of those roles, relationships, activities and facilities that might be relevant to a person. We argue that this should be based on the service user's wishes – what they want to do. However, it might be argued that other interested parties should be involved.
2 Identification of the person's strengths and assets that might be useful in gaining access to those roles, relationships, facilities and activities they desire.
3 Identification of those problems and disabilities that may impede access. In this context disabilities arising from three sources might be considered:
 a the mental health problems themselves
 b the way in which the person copes with, or has adapted to, their difficulties
 c the social disadvantages they experience.
 These disabling social disadvantages may be a consequence of mental health problems, e.g. poverty, loss of home, friends and family, unemployment and discrimination in a wide range of areas. They may also have predated mental health problems – things like childhood abuse, disrupted family relationships, poor

education – which left them with few personal, social and material resources with which to contend with their mental health difficulties (Wing and Morris, 1981).

4 Identification of relevant resources in the community: facilities, activities and supports available there.

Care planning within this model may employ a variety of interventions but all would be judged in terms of whether they facilitate access. Most crucially, a disability and access model shifts the focus from changing the individual to fit into the world to changing that world – by providing help, support and adaptation of that world – so that it can accommodate the person. For example, re-negotiation of work or family roles may be important so that the person is able to meet the demands of these roles. Similarly, access may be enhanced by providing support to other community agencies – colleges, leisure facilities, information and advice centres – and helping them to understand and accommodate people who experience serious mental health problems. This does not have to involve a grand scale 'educating the community' type of endeavour. Instead, it can be approached on an individual basis: advocating for an individual to attend classes or use particular facilities. Likewise, simple help and support in negotiating new situations, if necessary on an ongoing basis, may be important. However, the extent to which other people can usefully advocate for a disabled person is limited. At the bottom line, people with mental health problems are their own best advocates (Repper et al., 1997). The more that people with and without mental health problems can work, live and spend their leisure time alongside one another, the more barriers will be broken down. Clearly, developing skills and the reduction of some symptoms, or helping a person to cope with them better, may be of value in ensuring access but there are many other ways as well.

Who decides?

Probably the thorniest issue in relation to a problems-, needs- or disabilities-based perspective is: who determines what should be done? We have already discussed the numerous different stakeholders in the psychiatric enterprise: nowhere are their conflicting perspectives more evident than in the assessment of problems and needs or the determination of goals and methods of intervention. Central to all of these divergent interests is the relationship between the clinician and the service user.

Clinicians have traditionally had the deciding role: determining what should be done to the patient and how it should be done. This is justified on the basis of the specialist knowledge and expertise of the clinician. It is assumed that without the direction of the clinician, patients might make decisions that would not be in their best interests. The rise of the service user/survivor movement has seriously challenged this perspective (Chamberlin, 1977; O'Hagan, 1991; Campbell, 1996a,

1996b, 1996c) and there is now an increased emphasis on partnership both within services and in relation to decisions about individual care (Barker and Peck, 1996; Campbell, 1997).

Although much has undoubtedly changed, service users continue to express considerable dissatisfaction about services:

'Users suggest that the service has been developed and designed by professionals for users and that no matter how "empowered" users are in working with professionals they are still "passive recipients" of a model of care they find deeply unsatisfactory.' (Sainsbury Centre for Mental Health, 1997).

Service users argue that clinicians do not have a monopoly of experience and expertise. As a consequence of their personal experience of mental health problems and different interventions, and information they have gained from other users, they too have important expertise to bring to designing their own treatment and support. In addition, each user has their own ambitions, values and wishes which influence their treatment and support preferences. It is not the case that clinicians are being asked to give up their expertise, rather to use it in a different way:

'When mental health professionals are challenged by the survivor movement, they are being asked to change their relationship from one of paternalism to one of partnership.' (O'Hagan, 1991)

Such partnership can pose dilemmas for clinicians. Partnership is easy enough if clinician and service user fully discuss the different options available and both arrive at the same conclusion. Problems arise if they do not, and a reversion to paternalism is very tempting. As Mary O'Hagan goes on to say:

'My righteousness is always tempered by the sobering knowledge that if I had been a mental health worker instead of a survivor I would probably be all, or some, of the things I criticise them for.' (O'Hagan, 1991)

Real partnership and choice are not possible if users are denied the right to make decisions and adopt courses of action that the clinician does not consider best, and to receive support to pursue them. Clearly, there will be limits on this – like those imposed by mental health legislation – but these are relatively few and far between. All too often clinicians understandably wish to protect people from such things as failure, just as one might a child. For example, a person may wish to try to get a job or have a flat of their own, while the clinician may consider them unfit for work or independent living. At the bottom line, it is they who may fail and therefore it is they who should judge whether they wish to take this risk. If the clinician actively helps and supports the user in achieving their goal their chance of success is enhanced.

Values in community services

It is frequently the case that service users and clinicians have different ideas about what mental health services should be doing. These differences can cause major difficulties. If a service user's major interest is in getting their benefits sorted out or somewhere decent to live, while the clinician's primary concern is treating their delusional beliefs with medication or teaching them to cook, then a successful relationship is unlikely. If clinicians and users cannot agree on the primary issues to be addressed then user dissatisfaction is understandable.

In general, it is probably true to say that mental health services see their main role as treating mental illness. Traditionally this treatment would have almost exclusively taken the form of hospitalization and drugs or other physical therapy, but now it is increasingly supplemented by a range of psychological, psychoanalytic, arts, counselling, occupational and systemic therapies. At first sight this position seems relatively unproblematic: physical health services treat physical illness, mental health services treat mental illness. However, there are a number of difficulties in such parallels. A substantial proportion of those who use mental health services do not believe themselves to have a mental illness (Taylor and Perkins, 1991; Moodley and Perkins, 1991; Perkins and Moodley, 1993). Some people believe they have no problems at all, others believe their difficulties to be physical or social in nature, not psychiatric, and others believe that their unusual experiences are a valuable part of their lives which they do not wish to give up. If intervention solely involves treating people for illnesses they do not believe they have, or the symptoms of which they do not want to lose, good relationships are unlikely. Studies of what service users want from mental health services rarely indicate that treatment is a priority. Instead the ordinary things of everyday life take pride of place together with practical help and support.

Estroff (1993) looked at what mental health service users considered to be their unmet needs. The most common were: an adequate income, intimacy and privacy, a satisfying sex life, meaningful work, a satisfying social life, happiness, adequate resources and warmth. Service users typically say that services should provide better information and choice, be more accessible in providing help when and where it is needed, and in particular should *concentrate on practical help* including:

- *help with income and benefits*
- *help with finding employment*
- *help with housing and daily living skills*
- *counselling and advocacy*
- *practical support, such as child care*
- *help to access appropriate specialist services.*

(Sainsbury Centre for Mental Health, 1997)

Unfortunately, such practical assistance and support does not enjoy the same status in the eyes of providers as it does in those of users. Throughout mental health services, activities labelled 'therapy' or 'treatment' are highly valued while those labelled 'care' or 'support' have a lower status and often go almost unremarked. In an attempt to raise the status of some of these latter type of activities, there has been a tendency to give them 'therapy' or deceptively technical labels. So many leisure activities have been transformed into 'occupational therapy', cleaning one's room has become 'home management' and having a chat has been transformed into 'counselling'. Such a tendency may be understandable: these activities are important and their status should be recognized. However, to transform them into 'therapies' takes them out of the ordinary realm and endows them with a spurious specialism (Wolfensberger and Tullman, 1982).

What is needed instead is a revaluing of different components of care and a framework within which to understand them. The Sainsbury Centre for Mental Health, in their review of the future roles and training of mental health staff, argue that:

'... traditional training for mental health professionals has historically focused on "cure" rather than "care". This emphasis is no longer appropriate for work with people with severe mental illness... There is a need to develop models of long term care and support for this group and to train staff accordingly.' (Sainsbury Centre for Mental Health, 1997)

The provision of support and care is an art that requires skills which should not be underestimated. The skill is to provide help and support with things that most adults can do without infantilizing them or making them feel inadequate. Users quite frequently complain of '... offensive and patronising attitudes among staff' (Sainsbury Centre for Mental Health, 1997).

In avoiding such problems lessons can probably be learned from that help which is socially valued in our society. Service users should have as much control over the help as possible, when, where and how it is offered. 'Doing with' is often far more acceptable than 'doing for', but there are big individual differences in this regard and the person who is helped should direct the proceedings rather than the helper. Help should be presented in a manner which indicates that it is the individual's right to receive assistance, not an act of generosity on the part of the help giver. Finally, the helper must understand just how much more difficult it is to receive help than to give it. Giving help makes a person feel useful and valuable. Receiving help can all too easily make them feel useless and valueless and engender anger and resentment.

For people with ongoing mental health problems, a traditional 'illness and cure' approach is not useful. Repeated attempts at cure in the face of ongoing disability are not only futile and dispiriting to all concerned, they also detract attention from the very necessary task of helping the person to make the most of life with a disability. As we have discussed, a 'disability and access' approach may be far more appropriate. This would involve the shift in priorities that the Sainsbury Centre for Mental Health (1997) review demands. The aim of services would be to ensure that a person has access to those activities, facilities, roles and relationships they desire. Traditional interventions to minimize the distress caused by symptoms would still be necessary but equally, if not more important, would be practical support and help to enable people to gain access; assistance to gain and maintain the necessary money to do things; help to maintain housing and do what is necessary to live as independently as possible; help to find work and use community leisure facilities; help to find and make friends; support with the ups and downs of daily life. All of these would be central to providing care and *support in* communities and ensuring *access to* those communities. This is a reflection of what service users say they want from mental health services.

But is this the business of a health service? Health and social care

Enshrined in UK mental healthcare provision since the NHS and Community Care Act (DoH, 1990), is a distinction between 'health' and 'social' care: the former being the responsibility of health services, the latter of social services. The multiple needs of people who experience serious mental health problems clearly span this divide, posing numerous practical problems.

- There are simple co-ordination problems in ensuring seamless provision of care and support for an individual across multiple agencies.
- There is no clear distinction between what constitutes 'health' and 'social' care, and therefore that which is provided by different agencies is inconsistent from place to place, reflecting not the needs of service users but the historical balance of power and resources between agencies.
- Such unevenness can result in inequity. Healthcare remains (at the time of writing) free at the point of delivery, while social care does not have to be. Therefore, a person attending a health service day facility may get their lunch free while someone attending a social services facility may have to pay. Similarly, the different financial position of social services departments means that, for example, some make day centre users pay for their meals while others do not.
- In times of scarce resources, the absence of clarity concerning what constitutes 'health' and 'social' care makes it easier for everyone to declare that it is not their job – the health service deems it to be social care, social services say it is healthcare – and gaps in provision occur.

Underlying these difficulties is the problematic nature of the 'health' and 'social' care division. All 'disease', whether it be physical or psychiatric, has multiple causes and results from a complex interaction of physical, psychological, social and environmental events (Becker and Rosenstock, 1984). The distinction between 'health' and 'social' care is an economic or organizational one. It is nevertheless the case that such distinctions have been made and inter-agency working is a fact of life, not merely between health and social services but also with private and voluntary facilities, housing departments, employment agencies, education services and so forth. If access for people disabled by their mental health problems is to become a reality then it is not simply specialist mental health agencies who are involved. This diversity can pose huge dilemmas for clinicians: different agencies have different values, priorities and ways of working.

Working together to ensure that a person can gain access to the resources, facilities and services they want can be a time consuming affair and will raise questions about priorities: in the absence of increased resources, which of our existing activities can we give up in order to perform these new ones? Yet this is what users say they want from our services: advocacy and help to access appropriate services. It will almost certainly be time well spent. The opportunities that specialist mental health services can offer are necessarily limited, maybe one or two day centres, maybe one or two types of work. The community is a much wider sea of opportunity, offering numerous different types of work and activities, if we can render it accessible to service users (Rapp and Wintersteen, 1989).

Priorities

Decisions about what care and support should be provided are complex and they present clinicians with numerous dilemmas. Our assessments and care plans will critically depend upon the models we adopt. Are we trying to cure people of illnesses or help disabled people to make the most of their lives? Do we see 'throughput' as the goal? Is our aim to teach skills to service users so they can be more independent? If our focus is on meeting 'needs', then what do we mean by 'needs' and who should define them? Who should decide what we do? What should we be doing? Who should be doing what?

All too often such questions remain implicit rather than explicit and therefore end up as a nebulous source of friction between service users and different agencies. Any team or service must decide what it is trying to do and how it is trying to do it, and nowhere is this more critical than in relation to those people who have ongoing mental health problems; those who in the past have been consigned to the back wards, out of the sight of both communities and most clinicians, and whose problems remain despite psychiatry's attempts at cure. In moving from paternalism to partnership it is critical to adopt a model that is based on users' wants and wishes and offers hope and a positive way forward both for service users and those who support them.

9

Professional roles: blurring and differentiation

It is now widely accepted that a mental health team should be multi-disciplinary (Shepherd, 1990). The argument goes that, as people who experience serious mental health problems have multiple needs, so a variety of expertise is required to meet those needs. Typically a mental health team comprises psychiatrists, clinical psychologists, nurses, occupational therapists and social workers, but other therapists (art therapists, family therapists, psychotherapists, counsellors) might also be involved, as may legal and welfare rights advisors and advocates (Watts and Bennett, 1983; Perkins and Repper, 1996).

Each of these disciplines defines itself in terms of its core role, its expertise and its distinctive models or ways of understanding and intervening to alleviate problems (British Psychological Society, 1992; DoH, 1994c). Each has means of determining who may practice under its auspices via regulation of training, determination of codes of practice and systems of registration. Only those who have achieved the necessary training and practice requirements may call themselves a member of the profession, and they can be removed from the profession – 'struck off' – if they contravene the codes of practice or continuing training requirements.

Such regulation of a discipline is designed to maintain high standards of practice and make clear what can be expected of someone who is employed as a member of that profession. There are also benefits in terms of a clear status and identity for the individual professionals. The professional, service users and other staff know what is expected of them and what they can be asked to do. So a person who is experiencing problems with their medication knows that a psychiatrist may be the person to consult, while one with housing difficulties goes to the social worker. A recent study of users of a rehabilitation service revealed that they made clear distinctions between the role of different professionals: distinctions not dissimilar to those made by the professionals themselves (Meddings, 1997).

Despite the advantages of multi-professional teams, many difficulties can arise which cause dilemmas for practitioners.

The demarcation of professional skills

Rose (1989) has described how the mental sciences developed in the early nineteenth century to systematize, explain and thereby discipline and control that which had hitherto been considered below the level of description: ordinary, everyday individuality. Thus the mental sciences – psychiatry, psychology, psychoanalysis – began to describe what people were and how they could be changed. The theories, methods and techniques differed both within and across disciplines, but the 'individual' was for the first time invented as something which could be known in terms of the norms and values of the discipline. So, for example, in the case of psychoanalysis, human behaviour and experience started to be defined and understood within the framework of a variety of intrapsychic processes that were invented to explain why people thought, felt and behaved in the way that they did. Theories about how such intrapsychic processes operated were then used to predict and change people's thoughts, feelings and behaviour.

Yet none of the explanatory frameworks for defining and describing human behaviour and experience are 'objective facts'. Instead they represent different templates or models through which individuals can be viewed and their utility adjudged in terms of the extent to which they enable people to achieve control and reach their desired goals. For example, if a person wants to be able to cook then an understanding of their neurotransmitters or intrapsychic processes may not be particularly useful: instead an approach derived from learning theory may be preferable. If a person wants to work out a way of understanding what has happened to them, then a behavioural approach may not be the best.

There are, as ever, important questions to be asked concerning who should determine what is to be achieved, and thereby which model is most useful. If the aim is to minimize disruption in the community then quite different perspectives may be adopted than if the aim is to maximize community integration or user satisfaction with services. However, it must be emphasized that most models within the mental sciences can be used to achieve a variety of ends depending upon who is in control. The models developed by the mental health sciences have not remained within their disciplinary frameworks. They have seeped out into everyday language and constructions of the world so that many people think of themselves in various psychological and psychiatric terms: 'My mother was a nervous kind of person, I was born this way', 'It's my nerves', 'I've got low self-esteem'. It is not only professionals who have models for understanding human behaviour. Service users, as well as their relatives, friends and communities, also have ways of understanding experience and behaviour that are based on their own experiences, views and encounters with services (Pembroke, 1997).

Within the complicated abundance of professional and lay formulations of behaviour and experience, each profession endeavours to establish its uniqueness by demarcating that which is its own. Within any one discipline there are a number of different models adopted and as each discipline encompasses a broader range of models, so demarcation disputes with other disciplines are increased. For example, an occupational therapist may possess expertise in behaviourally-based skills training, while a clinical psychologist might claim behavioural models as his/her field of expertise. Alternatively, clinical psychologists, psychiatrists and specialist nurse therapists might all claim cognitive-behavioural approaches or family therapy as their own. Probably the only areas that remain within disciplinary boundaries are those strictly demarcated by legislation, e.g. the prescribing of medicine and decisions about compulsory detention in psychiatric hospital, and it seems unlikely that any discipline would choose to define its role solely in these terms.

Numerous problems can arise when different professionals, with overlapping skills, work together in multi-disciplinary teams: 'Who am I and what should I be doing?' 'If I do not do the things that make me a professional then I lose my identity.'

Loss of identity in community team settings is something about which many professionals have commented. For example, there have been disputes about whether anyone other than a consultant psychiatrist can be the 'team leader'. Psychiatrists in community mental health teams feel they have a lot more responsibility but not the corresponding authority, while in hospitals they were more likely to be regarded, by themselves and others, as the natural team leaders (Onyett *et al.*, 1995). Alternatively, Anciano and Kirkpatrick (1990) have discussed the difficulty in defining the 'specialist' nature of the clinical psychologist's role and feel that their identity is threatened by becoming part of community mental health teams. They question the wisdom of clinical psychologists 'giving away' their skills by training other disciplines. On the one hand they cite ethical considerations:

'... of other disciplines gaining a little knowledge and believing they are fully competent.'

On the other hand they cite economic considerations:

'... managers may look for ways of cutting back on staffing levels. If other staff begin to do our job then one can expect managers to question the uniqueness and usefulness of our profession ...'

The loss of identity, threat and feelings of isolation that result when someone is the sole representative of a profession within a multi-disciplinary team have been echoed by occupational therapists (Royal College of Psychiatrists and College of Occupational Therapists, 1992).

'Guild' disputes between professions for particular areas of work, while understandable in terms of preservation of identity, can only be destructive in relation to service provision. In particular, they can result in competition for those roles and tasks that cut across professions and are seen as having high status and a reluctance to engage in those which are perceived as having lower status. Service users can have little intrinsic interest in the status of the professionals who serve them. They require access to high quality services which provide the help and support they need in an acceptable manner, a requirement that is unlikely to be met by professionals battling among themselves about who should do what. The challenge is to enable professionals to maintain their identity while at the same time ensuring that all users' needs are met.

Professional skills and users' needs

There seems to be an unwritten assumption that multi-disciplinary teams are a 'good thing' and that a multi-professional group, working together, will automatically be able to meet the multi-faceted needs of the people whom they serve. Clearly, there are several problems with such assumptions. Whether or not the skills and expectations of professionals accord with the needs and wishes of service users is an empirical question. It is entirely possible that service users do not want what professionals want to do. Although the situation does not seem to be as grave as this, research does suggest some grounds for concern.

Shepherd et al. (1995) showed a level of agreement between professionals, service users and their relatives in relation to the importance of different elements of help and support, but they also found marked differences. Not surprisingly, professionals rated as most important those elements of care that most clearly reflected their own roles: treatment, symptom monitoring and professional support. Service users rated these things as significantly less important than more practical aspects of support. This clearly suggests the potential for conflict between users and professionals: professionals wishing to focus on treatment and monitoring, and users wanting assistance with the practicalities of life and living with mental health problems.

Such problems are likely to be aggravated by situations in which a desire to preserve professional identity results in inter-professional rivalries. These may take three forms:

1 Competition for those elements of help which have a high status among professionals (like treatment, therapy and symptom monitoring).
2 A reluctance to perform those professional tasks, like care planning, which may be expected of every discipline. Although all might agree that the proper co-ordination

and documentation of help and support is essential, pressure of work and the fact that tasks like care planning do not specifically fall within the remit of any profession can lead to everyone passing the buck.

3 A failure to perform tasks that are not really considered 'professional' tasks at all. Many of the things which people want and need of services – especially practical, day-to-day assistance – do not fall within the core role definition of any traditional mental health professional and are often considered to be 'menial' tasks that lower one's status ('I'm a nurse, not a cleaner', 'It's not a psychologist's job to take someone to work'). Who should wash socks? Does it really take six years of training to wield a vacuum cleaner?

In resolving such questions, a critical starting point revolves around the relative value accorded different jobs. Most professionals were trained within a 'treatment' or 'cure'-based paradigm: the aim being to intervene to eliminate or minimize a person's problems. Within such a paradigm it is hardly surprising that the elements of help that they most value are treatment and symptom monitoring (whether this be medical, psychological or psychotherapeutic). However, when a person has ongoing disabilities as a consequence of their mental health problems, then such a cure perspective becomes less useful (Ekdawi and Conning, 1994; Perkins and Repper, 1996). Instead, a paradigmatic shift is required to look at how people can best be assisted to live with, and make the most of life with, their disabilities. Such a shift does not render traditional treatments (of whatever genre) redundant, rather it renders them relatively less important. Support in the practicalities of everyday life with a disability and help in adjusting to what this means take on a higher profile. Service users have recognized these relative priorities (Shepherd et al., 1995; Sainsbury Centre for Mental Health, 1997) and it is important that professionals also recognize the change and begin to accord higher value to such areas.

The lower value attached to supporting people in practical tasks is based on the implicit assumption that they are in some way easier and do not require the extensive training and experience that most professionals receive. It is probably true to say that most professional training does not prepare its trainees to provide practical help, but the provision of such support certainly does require considerable skill (Perkins and Repper, 1996). First, there is the delicate balance to be reached between providing too much help and too little. If too much help is provided, then the person is unable to use the skills they have (and risks losing them) and is also made to feel less confident in their abilities – 'If the staff are doing this for me then what I am able to do must be no good.' If too little help is provided then the person is not able to cope and may well feel even more incompetent because they have to ask for more assistance – 'They expect me to be able to do these things, otherwise they would have given me more help. But I can't so I'm obviously more useless than they think.'

Allied with this is the provision of the correct kind of help. People with serious mental health problems are not globally incompetent. Rather, because of their cognitive and emotional difficulties, there may be some elements of tasks that are difficult and these may cause the whole task performance to break down. For example, a person who is unable to shop for themselves may have problems in a variety of areas. They may have difficulty in planning what they want to eat and deciding what to buy, in which case help with drawing up shopping lists may be needed but not help with actually going to the shop. Alternatively, they may have difficulty going into a crowded shop because they believe everyone is looking at them, in which case they may need help in actually going and doing the shopping but not planning what to buy. Or perhaps the person could gain a greater degree of independence by going regularly to less crowded local shops rather than to large supermarkets. Perhaps they can gradually develop some of the skills needed and become less dependent on staff, perhaps they cannot. Perhaps they only need help when they are having a bad time with their symptoms, in which case careful plans are needed to give them the assistance they need only when they require it. Providing each individual with exactly the right type and amount of help when they need it can be an extremely skilled affair requiring a detailed knowledge of the person, their needs, preferences and problems.

Finally, a high level of interpersonal skill is required to deliver help in an acceptable manner. People who experience serious mental health problems often require assistance with tasks that it is assumed most adults can do unaided. It is understandable, and not uncommon, for people to experience assistance as belittling and infantilizing: many complain about staff treating them like children. Unless practical help can be provided in a manner that preserves the dignity and pride of the person receiving it then that person may well refuse the assistance they need. In this context there are probably two general principles that are important. First, the person has a *right* to receive assistance. Second, the person should have as much *control* over that assistance as possible.

But who should actually do it?

Given that the provision of day-to-day help is so essential and requires considerable sensitivity and skill, it is important that such areas take a central role in multi-disciplinary assessment and care planning: not in broad general terms ('assist with self-care') but with the same specificity as monitoring of mental state or particular treatments are considered. If the proper team consideration is accorded to all areas of intervention – including practical help and those needs which fall outside the core role of any profession – then their status can be raised. All professions will be involved in deciding what is done even if they are not involved in the delivery of assistance.

However, there remains the question of who should provide those aspects of care – like care planning and day-to-day help – that fall outside the core role of any profession? There can be no absolute answers and local circumstances may be important. Where particular professionals are more numerous than others then it will be possible for them to take on more of the tasks which are outside the traditional role of all professions. However, as the more numerous professions are often those with the historically lower status in mental health services, especially nurses, this can aggravate existing inter-professional rivalries. If nurses are required to do all those tasks which are currently deemed 'low status' (but in fact require considerable skill) then this may make them feel even further devalued. If, in understandable response, they feel 'put upon' by other disciplines, then the service provided to users suffers. Either 'low status' tasks will not be done or they will be done reluctantly and in a manner that makes users feel bad for requiring the help.

The professional expertise of most disciplines may well be relevant in areas well outside their traditional remit. For example, in relation to practical assistance, psychiatrists might have useful contributions to make in their understanding of psychopathology, the effects of medication and the relationship between these and the areas in which performance is likely to break down. Clinical psychologists have access to a variety of models of psychological functioning and psychopathology which can also inform the process of providing practical help, and both they and occupational therapists have expertise in the assessment of performance, the identification of specific areas in which performance has broken down and skills training. Social workers have access to a wealth of information about resources available and ways in which needs can be met using facilities available in the local community.

Although the provision of practical help may be seen as being outside the core role of any professional, different professionals may be able to bring useful intelligence to bear in these traditionally extra-professional areas. However, they will all be handicapped in using this expertise if they never actually provide the help on which they are advising. Therefore it would seem necessary that everyone has at least some experience of providing practical help: of helping a person to wash their socks. At a more practical level, there are likely to be some users who have a particularly good relationship with one professional rather than another, and will only accept help from that person. In such instances it would seem simply churlish if this professional refused the help because it was not their job.

While all disciplines may have a role to play in relation to providing those aspects of care and support which fall outside traditional roles, questions also arise about the extent to which professionals are necessary for performing many aspects of care. If it is not a professional's job then why employ professionals? It could be argued that those tasks which do not strictly require professional expertise should not be performed by professionals. If they are it is not only wasteful of expensive training, but risks professionalizing the ordinary. Everyday tasks, such as vacuum cleaning, cutting toe nails and chatting to someone, suddenly fall outside the realm of competence of most people and require years of training. If all aspects of helping and interacting with distressed and disabled people are seen as 'professional' tasks then the prospect of integration in communities further recedes. On the other hand, if professionals never engage with the ordinary lives of those whom they serve and deal only with pathological elements that relate to their professional expertise, how can they know them? How can they plan treatment and support that is relevant to the whole person? How can they help them to develop their strengths and rebuild their lives? It seems likely that a balance is required between professional engagement with the whole person and avoidance of rendering 'professional' that which is not.

There are now a number of services that have employed non-professionally qualified staff to assist in the provision of care and support. A variety of mental health support workers, mental healthcare assistants, occupational therapy assistants, psychology assistants and psychiatry clinical assistants are involved in providing treatment and care. Some, like assistant psychologists and psychiatry clinical assistants, are required to have qualifications (but not in mental health), others need not. The most numerous of these non-professionally qualified workers are the mental health support workers and mental healthcare assistants who have been employed to provide practical and emotional support to users in a variety of services.

The employment of non-professionally qualified staff to do some of the tasks that fall outside the remit of professional staff can have advantages. Such people can focus on the provision of ordinary help and support which does not require professional training and which professionals do not have the resources to perform. If they are properly supervised then the skills of professionals can be used (where necessary) to good effect in guiding the work of their non-professional colleagues, and the workforce can be enhanced by a greater range of skills and experience. On the negative side, a situation can result where the majority of direct contact with service users is with non-professionally qualified staff. This could potentially decrease the skills directly available to service users. There is also a potential threat to professionals: if most of the support that service users need does not require professionally trained staff then the number of professionals might be reduced. However, since it is often the case that difficulties are experienced in recruiting trained professionals (Sainsbury Centre for Mental Health, 1997), such threats may be more theoretical than real. Nevertheless, it behoves any profession to examine precisely which aspects of its work really require 'professional' training and which could be equally well, if not better, performed by non-professionally qualified, specifically trained staff.

Clearly, issues of training non-professionally qualified staff become important and are an arena that offers both opportunities and problems. It has been difficult to find, at a national level, appropriate training programmes and many services have found the available National Vocational Qualifications inadequate to their needs. The development of separate training and induction programmes in each local area may be less than efficient, but it ensures that staff are equipped for the jobs required of them. The tailoring of training to local staff needs offers opportunities to target the skill mix within the team and develop a certain flexibility in response to users' needs and local circumstances.

In this context issues relating to who is best equipped to perform the necessary training are particularly important. While traditional professionals may have something to offer, the provision of practical help does not fall within their core role. Perhaps those best equipped to perform at least a substantial part of training of support workers might be service users themselves. Service users are, after all, the experts on the effectiveness of different ways of providing help and support and an increasing number of user trainers are now available to share this expertise with staff. Service users' expertise can also be used in staff training in other ways. For example, in the rehabilitation and continuing care service in which one of the authors works, several service users complained about the way in which staff (many of whom were mental health support workers) treated them (Perkins, 1997). The Service Users' Forum produced a list of things which they found offensive or demeaning, this was then circulated to all staff and used

- in one-to-one supervision
- in the introductory training for the service
- in more general 'customer care' training.

In relation to existing professionals, major changes in the existing 'guilds' seem unlikely to occur. However, the review conducted by the Sainsbury Centre for Mental Health (1997) has recommended some changes. In particular, it has suggested that a series of 'core competencies' – skills necessary in all mental health professionals – be established and developed through shared learning and inter-professional education. Within each profession there should be occupational standards linked to the core competencies. This would go some way to extending the core role definition of each profession and formalize the overlap between them, thereby making a variety of tasks and skills the responsibility of all. Further, the Sainsbury Centre for Mental Health (1997) review recommended that, in the training of all professionals:

'options for encouraging user and carer involvement in curriculum planning, training delivery and setting service standards relating to continued fitness for purpose and assessment of competence should be developed and implemented.'

The multi-faceted nature of mental healthcare and support

Typically, consideration of the staff who should comprise a mental health team begins with an assumption that certain professions must be represented – psychiatry, clinical psychology, occupational therapy, nursing and social work – and then the required numbers and grades of each considered. While this may be understandable given the present structure of services and the different professional interest groups, it may not be the best approach. A better starting point must surely be the needs of those people whom the service is designed to serve. Shepherd *et al.* (1995), on the basis of both previous research and clinical practice, identified 11 such areas of need:

1 Professional support and continuity of care.
2 Clear information to users and carers regarding 'illness', symptoms, outcome and factors affecting the likelihood of further breakdowns.
3 Help to come to terms with the 'illness' via personal counselling to help the person make sense of their problems.
4 Stable, good-quality housing and/or direct help with housekeeping tasks (shopping, cooking etc.).
5 Access to basic financial and material support (benefit entitlements etc.) and/or help with money management.
6 Adequate and meaningful daytime activities (work, leisure, social activities etc.).
7 Social support at home where the residential setting is shared by others (e.g. family homes or sheltered accommodation) including 'expressed emotion' issues with respect to family and non-family carers.
8 Access to an appropriate network of social support outside the home in line with the person's wishes.
9 Effective treatment of symptoms while minimizing side-effects, including medication, psychological approaches and other therapies.
10 Monitoring of changes in symptoms on a regular basis, early detection of signs of relapse and planning for the management of acute crises.
11 Maintaining good physical health.

All of these achieved a mean rating of at least 'important' by a group of 162 professionals, 143 users and 112 family carers. It is very difficult to map on to the above list the role of the specific professions. It is not possible to say, for example, that items 1–3 are the job of the psychiatrist, 4–6 the social worker and so forth. Instead, many of the needs could be met by the skills that a variety of professionals possess, others do not seem to require professional skills at all and yet others may require expertise that is not part of the core role of any mental health profession. In short, it does not appear that existing professional distinctions readily map on to users' needs. If expertise were recruited in relation to such needs the composition of teams might look very different.

   In this context, the structure of community support teams for people with serious ongoing mental health problems in the USA is of interest (Perkins, 1993). Such teams are particularly noteworthy because many of the models of good practice adopted in the UK were developed from the North American experience (Stein and Test, 1980). With some notable exceptions (like the PACT team in Madison, Wisconsin) it is rare in the USA for a psychiatrist to lead a community care service: typically they would have sessional input designed solely to monitor medication and mental state. In all cases, even where the psychiatrist is the team leader, the remainder of the team would comprise generic 'case managers' without the typical UK requirements for so many nurses, psychologists etc. All case managers must have at least a master's degree in a relevant discipline but they would be recruited on the basis of their specific skills and the needs of the team. Thus, if the team is short of family therapists, a case manager with family therapy qualifications would be recruited irrespective of their discipline. Typically, teams are comprised of a mixture of psychiatric nurses (a masters degree level qualification in the USA), social workers and psychologists from a variety of specialities (not usually clinical psychologists, but often rehabilitation or occupational psychologists). This approach moves away from the traditional 'guilds' of the UK while at the same time ensuring a high level of professional competence and a flexibility that could be used to ensure the team had within it all the necessary skills.

In the more restrictive UK context, it is important to remember that professionals bring with them far more than the skills of their profession. Watts and Bennett (1983) have suggested that team members bring three attributes:

1 the core skills of their discipline
2 specialized post-qualification skills and experience (e.g. family therapy, work with seriously disabled people)
3 different life experiences and social backgrounds.

Perhaps it is time to place at least as much stress on the latter attributes as the former one. Post-qualification training and experience may not be discipline-specific but may greatly enhance the range of skills available within the team. By seeking or funding the acquisition of such qualifications it may be possible to actively construct teams that more accurately reflect the skills required to meet the needs of their users.

Life experiences can be of central importance. These may include general characteristics such as race, culture and class as well as specific interests and skills such as football or DIY (essential if one is helping someone to set up home). For example, we know one man who spent almost all his time in bed, despite the skilled endeavours of many trained professionals, until a young – non-professionally qualified – male member of staff joined the team. This man had two interests – football (Chelsea) and religion – which coincided with those of the user, and was himself a service user. It was not long before they had formed an excellent working relationship and the service user was going out regularly, with and without his new-found ally. Staff may also bring personal experiences of mental health problems, either as users of mental health services or as carers, which can enhance their abilities and understanding (Davidson and Perkins, 1997).

The core skills of each profession may be necessary for the provision of effective treatment and support, but they are not sufficient. A range of non-profession-specific skills are required, together with skills that do not fall within the remit of any traditional mental health professions. The attitude, personal characteristics and background of staff will also be critical to their effectiveness, and it seems likely that many tasks can be performed by non-professionally qualified people. It is perhaps time to stop saying 'we need a psychiatrist, a clinical psychologist, an occupational therapist and a nurse' and to start looking at the needs of service users and at who can best meet these.

10

Users, relatives and professionals

Serious mental health difficulties have a profound impact not only on the life of the individual who experiences them, but also on the lives of those around them (WHO, 1965). The difficulties experienced by the relatives of those who are disabled by mental health problems have been widely documented (Creer *et al.*, 1982; Willis, 1982; Gibbons *et al.*, 1984; Fadden *et al.*, 1987; Shepherd *et al.*, 1994, 1995). Relatives often feel that staff blame the family for the person's difficulties and feel relatively unsupported and ill-informed by services. As well as coping with numerous practical difficulties, they understandably experience complex emotional responses:

'Grief is a key reaction experienced by many relatives of persons with serious mental illness. Parents, spouses, and children may endure great longing for the quality of their former relationship with the ill person, as well as grief over dashed hopes and aspirations.' (Miller, 1996)

However, in a study of 125 families, Doll (1976) found that, despite heavy social and emotional strains, they looked after their disabled relative without shame or distress. In a similar fashion, Fadden *et al.* (1987) found that families tended to understate the degree of hardship with which they had to contend.

Relationships between the individual and their relatives, friends, acquaintances and colleagues necessarily change if a person's circumstances alter and they are no longer able to meet former expectations. It is the sad fact that many more peripheral relationships may be lost. However, new relationships can be forged as a consequence of the person's problems, often with others who experience similar difficulties, and other relationships with family and close friends may intensify in positive ways, not simply negative ones.

Research has shown that relatives want acknowledgement from professionals of their role as carers; recognition of their value as partners in care; increased access to professional support; information about the illness and regular updates from professionals; improved service co-ordination; better communication with professionals; and opportunities to learn coping strategies (Shepherd et al., 1994; Sainsbury Centre for Mental Health, 1997). While such requests may, at first sight, seem reasonable, it is not uncommon for the wishes and interests of service users and their relatives to diverge – a divergence which can pose dilemmas for professionals.

Users and carers

It has become commonplace within mental health services to hear talk of involving and ascertaining the views of 'users and carers'. (DoH, 1995a; Clinical Standards Advisory Group, 1995). This conjunction of users and carers as a single interest group is problematic. It is important to recognize that, while users and their relatives may share some common interests and concerns, there is no necessary reason why they should do so. In many areas, their views, priorities and preferences may well be different (Shepherd et al., 1994; 1995). Irrespective of the quality of their family relationships, there can be very few adults who would wholly share the views and aspirations of their parents or who would want them to speak on their behalf on all issues. Adults with serious mental health problems are no different. This is not to say that the views and concerns of relatives are unimportant, they are not, but they may be different from those of service users (just as the views of professionals, local communities, the police and so forth may be) and should be treated as such.

The bracketing together of users and carers can easily become a way of ignoring the views of those who experience serious mental health problems. Carers may not experience such difficulties which can mean that they are better able to participate in mental health planning and service systems. It is easier for purchasers, planners and professionals to include relatives who may be more articulate and insistent than their disabled kinfolk. In addition, the temptation to interpret what service users say as a manifestation of their disabilities may increase this tendency to pay heed to the views of relatives rather than service users. If users and carers are considered to be a single entity then, in involving relatives, services may erroneously consider themselves to have consulted service users.

Relatives, carers and the 'burden of care'?

As in the phrase 'users and carers', there is a tendency to define relatives as 'carers' or 'informal carers'. Undoubtedly this terminology would be justified on the basis that some informal carers are not relatives. However, it remains the case that the vast majority of people referred to as 'carers'/'informal carers' are in fact relatives, usually parents, and if a broader category were required then a phrase like 'relatives and friends' could be adopted.

The way in which roles and relationships are labelled matters as it defines their quality and value. The change in terminology from 'relative' or 'friend' to 'carer' has important implications. The term relative refers to a whole host of kinship, social and emotional connections and reciprocal responsibilities as does the term 'friend'. To be a relative or a friend is to enjoy a reciprocity and a form of equality: the precise roles may vary (mother/sister) but the status (relative) is the same. Such reciprocity is reflected in semantic as well as relational terms and, in both cases, the other party in the relationship is also a 'relative' or a 'friend'.

In changing our construction from 'relative' to 'carer' this reciprocity and equality is lost. The other party in the relationship is not a 'carer', they are the 'cared for'. Here there is a clear hierarchy of competence and the more competent 'carer' looks after the less competent 'cared for'. This type of construction has encouraged:

- The development of an extensive research literature concerning the 'burden of care' imposed on families living with a relative who is seriously disabled by mental health problems (Creer et al., 1982; Goldman, 1982; Thompson and Doll, 1982; Gibbons et al., 1984; Fadden et al., 1987; Cook and Pickett, 1987; Lefley, 1989; Marsh, 1992).
- The development of instruments for measuring this burden (Scheme et al., 1994, reviewed some 21 different measures of family burden).
- The expression of surprise by several researchers and clinicians when families do not complain of this 'burden' in the manner they think the 'objective' situation warrants (Doll, 1976; Fadden et al., 1987).

While in no way wishing to minimize the pressures on family members and friends, including the disabled person him/herself, there are a number of problems in moving to a construction of relatives as 'carers' and the associated exploration and evaluation of the 'burden of care'. It is oppressive and devaluing to the disabled person him/herself. They are the incompetent 'cared for', they are the 'burden' on their family and friends: hardly a positive and affirming position. People who experience serious mental health problems have many skills, assets and abilities – things that they can contribute to their families – that are lost if they become simply a 'burden of care'. Szmukler (1996) in a critique of the concept of family 'burden' argues that:

'Carers' problems are now usually framed in terms of "burden", a term which I believe hinders our thinking about the processes involved... More than being simply unhelpful... the term "burden" is pejorative, connoting a passive load borne by carers... In an era when patients are encouraged to participate actively in their own care, the inertia implied by the term is offensive... it restricts carers' reactions to the negative. Rewarding aspects of caregiving and valued aspects of the relationship with the patient are excluded even though carers, if asked, commonly report them.'

Although roles and relationships may change this does not have to mean that these are any less valued. As two fathers said of their sons with serious mental health problems:

'I'd always expected him to get married and leave home, but as it is we're lucky to still have him around. We have always enjoyed bird watching together and now we can go whenever we like.'

'I'm so proud of him. He was so ill, and now look – he's out every day working at the centre and he runs errands for me – I can't get up and down those stairs very well now, you know.'

Unfortunately, a focus on 'burden' has lead to a dearth of research on the positive contribution that people with mental health problems can make to their families. We could find only a single research paper examining this issue (Greenberg *et al.*, 1994). The authors argue that:

'Over the past four decades, studies have largely focused on the burdens families experience... because research to date has focused on the role of the patient as recipient of care and support, we have a major gap in our knowledge about the positive roles played by persons with serious mental illness.'

In a large study of a broad cross-section of 725 people with serious mental health problems and their families, they found that users, especially those who lived with their families, played positive roles within those families. According to their families they provided substantial practical and emotional help to their relatives: between 50 and 80% helped by doing household chores, shopping, listening to problems, providing companionship and providing news about family and friends.

From this research it is clear that the relationship between people with serious mental health problems and their families cannot be reduced to one of 'carer' and 'cared for'. Such a limited vision masks the continuing, and reciprocal, love, affection and support that can exist within families when a member is disabled. Many people with serious mental health problems in the Greenberg *et al.* (1994) study were providing a listening ear and emotional support to their relatives, looking after them when they were ill and providing practical help. Roles and relationships within families may have changed, and may have deviated from the prior expectations of all parties in a distressing manner. But the ensuing roles and relationships were not of 'carer' and 'cared for': care was something done by all parties, but their relationships were richer and more complex than this.

Finally, the translation of relatives into carers means that those relatives who are not carers are disenfranchised. The majority of people with serious mental health problems do not live with their relatives. In their survey of 725 families, Greenberg *et al.* (1994) found that in only 23.7% did the disabled relative live with their family. In an inner London borough as few as 10% of the nearly 900 people in long-term contact with mental health services lived with their relatives (Perkins and Twelftree, 1997). Different patterns of population mobility mean that this figure varies – for example in Sheffield, 40% of people in contact with community mental health nurses lived with relatives (Brooker and Conway, 1995). However, many people remain very much a part of their families even when their family is not their carer. Failure to recognize the importance of relationships within families who do not live together has led to research into family interventions focusing only on those families who do live together (Leff *et al.*, 1982; Falloon *et al.*, 1984; Dixon and Lehman, 1995). It has also sometimes led to a failure to consult and involve relatives and friends who, while not direct carers, may be very important to the disabled person.

Families and professionals

We have already described some of the difficulties that arise in relationships between service users and professionals. It is also the case that relationships between professionals and relatives have been problematic. Relatives often feel blamed for the person's mental health problems, complain that professionals do not listen to them or involve them in treatment planning, and say that they do not receive enough support, especially at times of crisis (Willis, 1982; Holden and Levine, 1982; Shepherd *et al.*, 1994, 1995; Fadden *et al.*, 1987; Petrila and Sadoff, 1992). Based on information from both relatives and clinicians, Winefield and Burnett (1996) have suggested a series of barriers to relative–professional relationships. These all pose dilemmas for clinicians and will be used as the framework for discussion here.

Conflicts between professionals' relationships with relatives and service users

Professionals have a primary responsibility to the service user, but the nature of their relationship with the person's family is less clear: whose responsibility is the well-being of relatives? Given the potential for conflicting interests, it might be preferable if relatives received support from an entirely different service (or at least different professionals within the same service) so that divided loyalties might to some extent be avoided. However, this may not always be possible and many difficulties would still remain.

Many of the dilemmas that arise for clinicians stem directly from a struggle for power and the fact that professionals, service users and their relatives have different views, priorities and concerns. Confidentiality problems can arise in which the clinician is directly caught between the interests of the service user and those of the relative (Atkinson and Coia, 1989; Petrila and Sadoff, 1992). The clinician is obliged to respect a person's wishes not to keep their relatives informed, but this can cause huge rifts in relationships between staff and relatives. If a service user goes to stay with their partner, or stops taking medication, or gets pregnant and does not want their family to know, or simply does not want relatives involved in their care plan, then relatives can feel understandably betrayed, excluded and ill-informed about things which may directly affect them.

Situations can arise when conflicts occur between the service user and their relatives and staff are required to 'side' with one or other party. Such differences may relate to the ordinary developmental issues that challenge most families in late adolescence – sex, drink, drugs, 'acceptable' behaviour – but they can also revolve around issues concerning the person's mental health problems. If, for example, a person's parents believe that they are 'getting worse' and the person does not, then professionals have to make judgements about who they will believe. Whichever choice is made, the 'disbelieved' party is likely to feel let down and relationships worsen. Such conflicts of interest can come to a head in relation to compulsory hospitalization and treatment: the civil rights of the service user versus the needs (and even safety) of their relatives.

Parents perceived as responsible for the illness

It is unsurprising that families feel blamed by professionals for a relative's mental health problems. The idea that parents might be responsible for schizophrenia (and other serious mental health problems) dates back to a post-Second World War era in which there was a desire to move away from biological models of aetiology. All the early models were essentially cognitive, arguing that adverse early experience led to ways of perceiving and interacting with the social world that corresponded to the symptoms of schizophrenia. The concept of the schizophrenogenic mother was suggested by Fromm-Reichman in 1948. Lidz and Lidz (1949) reported two types of abnormal family pattern – marital skew and marital schism – in families with one member who had been given a diagnosis of schizophrenia. By 1956, Bateson and his colleagues had formulated the theory that schizophrenia resulted from the 'double bind' communication within families. Wynne and Singer (1963) believed schizophrenia to result from a fragmented or amorphous parenting style, and Laing and Esterson (1964) held that schizophrenia was an understandable response to the pressures in the family and society at large.

Although such theories have been widely criticized and empirical evidence to support them does not exist (Hirsch and Leff, 1975), it appears that many mental health professionals continue to adhere to their underlying ideas and continue to believe that in some way families cause schizophrenia. Such ideas have been reinforced by two factors. First, many people with serious mental health problems have experienced sexual and physical abuse. This has fuelled concern about the adult consequences of abuse in childhood and the role that this may have in the problems of those with serious mental health difficulties (Williams and Watson, 1994). Even if such abuse is not considered causal of major mental health problems *'it may cause professionals to feel angry with parents'* (Winefield and Burnett, 1996).

Second, although research into the causal link between patterns of interaction in the family and schizophrenia may have largely ceased, families have been implicated in causing relapse, most notably in relation to the influential concept of 'high expressed emotion'. Brown *et al.* (1958) found that, contrary to their expectations, patients who returned to live with their parents or spouses after hospitalization fared relatively badly. Noting that this effect depended on the amount of contact between the person and their relatives, they tentatively suggested that certain intense relationships might increase risk of relapse. This led to a series of studies spanning two decades and the birth of the concept of 'high expressed emotion' (Brown and Rutter, 1966; Brown *et al.*, 1972; Vaughn and Leff, 1976; Vaughn and Leff, 1981; Ferrera and Vizarro, 1988). A composite measure of 'high expressed emotion' in terms of 'emotional over-involvement' and a high level of 'critical comments' on the part of relatives (usually parents), combined with a high level of face-to-face contact (in excess of 35 hours per week), was found to predict relapse.

Despite the enthusiasm for ideas of expressed emotion and the therapeutic interventions it has spawned (Leff *et al.*, 1982, 1985), it remains the case that families are 'blamed', if not for causing the problems in the first place, then for causing relapses. As Winefield and Burnett (1996) describe, if professionals blame relatives for the person's problems, then the relative has a series of unenviable choices:

- *accept the professional's view about their own causal role in the patient's illness and feel depressed and guilty*
- *reject the professional's view and become angry and alienated from the therapist*
- *waver in confusion and suffer both guilt and alienation.*

Hatfield *et al.* (1987), in their critique of the theory of 'high expressed emotion' (EE) and its associated research, argue that:

'EE is not enough of a departure from traditional theories that blamed families for mental illness to overcome families' alienation from the mental health profession. Since high EE is seen as undesirable, then high EE families may justifiably feel that they have been labelled "bad families". Once again, the focus is on family deficit and families are viewed negatively. Professionals seem unaware of the depth of family caring, the persistence of family members in the face of incredible odds, their creativity and inventiveness, and their heroic efforts to aid their family member when there is little positive in his or her life. There is, perhaps, more to be learned from studying the strengths of people rather than their frailties. It is upon their strengths that alliances with professionals can be built.'

Unless professionals are able to view relatives and friends of a service user in a positive light and as a resource that the service user has, it seems unlikely that effective relationships can ever be formed.

Relatives' lack of gratitude to professionals

Winefield and Burnett (1996) found that relatives' lack of gratitude towards staff, combined with their anger and complaints about services provided, was a further factor mitigating against good relationships between staff and relatives:

'Participants agreed with the fact of relatives' ingratitude... citing "the extremely minimal number of boxes of chocolates received in psychiatric wards compared with medical and surgical wards".'

The problem in this context is not relatives' lack of gratitude, but clinicians' expectations of gratitude. Many professionals expect to be thanked for their efforts and this can be a problem. It is interesting to note that Perkins and Repper (1996) described how professionals' expectations of gratitude for their efforts are a barrier to forming effective relationships with service users: they may be a similar barrier to relationships with relatives and friends of service users. In this context it is important to consider how staff receive support and praise for their work within teams and services in a way that does not require them to seek it from service users. Professionals are, after all, employed to meet the needs of users of the service, not the other way around.

Conflicts and anxieties over power

Conflicts over power – who decides? who knows best? – are a theme running through most dilemmas that arise for clinicians, and relationships with relatives are no exception. Staff members in Winefield and Burnett's (1996) study feared loss of professional power if they shared information with relatives. They were also concerned that if relatives were fully involved, professional ignorance, shortcuts and mistakes might be revealed.

Just as a service user develops an understanding and knowledge of their own problems that is far more extensive than that of professionals, so relatives/friends often know a great deal about a service user. As with many people in long-term relationships, years of intimacy teaches how things might best be done: what the person likes and does not like, what upsets them, how best to help them do the things they want to do and so forth. Professionals typically have a much more circumscribed knowledge of the person. However, in acknowledging relatives' and friends' expertise, like acknowledging the expertise of service users, their power is reduced.

Deficiencies in professional training and resources

Human resources constitute the largest component of any mental health system, and staff training and expertise are important. Professionals in the Winefield and Burnett

(1996) study felt that they had not received training in the group and family therapy skills necessary to simultaneously form alliances with both the service user and their relatives. Such lack of training and expertise has been remarked by others (Clinical Standards Advisory Group, 1995; DoH, 1994c). The absence of training and understanding of a family's situation can lead to negative stereotyping of relatives and avoidance of interacting with families and friends. Other barriers to forming effective relationships with families might lie in more practical areas (Winefield and Burnett, 1996). It is important to make time to listen to the views of relatives and friends. Trying to form effective relationships with both individual service users and the people who are important to them, then attempting to consult all and resolve the difficulties of each, requires considerable professional time and skill.

In essence, clinicians typically walk a narrow tightrope in a three-way tussle for power: the interests of the service user, their relatives and friends and what the clinician thinks is best. From a traditional, systemic family therapy perspective it is not the individual service user but the whole family who are considered to be the patient (Campbell and Draper, 1985) thus avoiding (or obscuring) differences between the person and their family except in so far as these are part of the overall family dynamics. Although professionals have a primary responsibility towards the users of their services, it cannot be in a service user's interests to alienate those people who are important to them. In so far as the individual has or wishes to have access to them, relatives constitute an important social resource. If these relatives are alienated by a mental health service that excludes them, blames them for the person's problems or fails to support them, then it is the service user who is the ultimate loser. A balance between according pride of place to the interests of the service user, while at the same time engaging and supporting their relatives, is essential. However, in this context, it may be important to look to broader social networks than simply 'family'.

Beyond parents: siblings, lovers, friends...

In most considerations of the social context of people who experience serious mental health problems the family reigns supreme, especially parents and spouses. While it is undoubtedly the case that parents and spouses provide a great deal of love and support, there are many other people in an individual's world who may be equally, if not more, important. For example, as with any other adults, siblings can be central in the lives of service users, but there is a dearth of literature concerning their role and the problems they face. In one of the few studies that exists, Titelman (1991) found the dominating themes in the experience of siblings of people with a diagnosis of schizophrenia to be: protracted mourning, guilt because they had not developed schizophrenia ('survivor' guilt) and fear of madness in themselves and identification with their disabled sibling. Despite such difficulties, it is rare for services to address their needs specifically and more often than not they remain shadowy figures in the background if 'closer' relatives (parents, spouses) exist.

Beyond the immediate nuclear family, the literature appears to dry up completely. There is nothing about the experience of the broader family network which may be particularly important in some cultures. Neither do non-married partners or lesbian/ gay partners feature in writings about the kin of people with serious mental health problems. Similarly, the value of, and difficulties experienced by, friends of the disabled person have received little attention. Too often, the friends of someone who experiences serious mental health problems simply drift away over the years until they have little or no contact with people they knew before their problems began. It is interesting to speculate whether such a drift could be reduced if professionals actively involved and included close friends of the person's choice.

There is evidence from the writings of service users that friends – both those who were known before a person's problems began and those who they have met since – can be extremely important.

'I have several times been involved in situations where friends, flatmates and relatives have decided to support someone in crisis to stay out of hospital or, at least, shorten their stay. A degree of organization has proved useful. On one occasion, five of us set up a rota to visit a colleague (I'll call her Jean) who was being held under section. Two of us went each day to spend an hour or so listening to her. Once a week, the group met to share our thoughts and fears about the situation. Jean was able to leave hospital far sooner than the staff had predicted, and our meetings had prepared us and her well for her return to the house where most of us lived. It wasn't easy. We were stretched and stressed out. But we all felt we had learnt a lot from the experience. We felt closer to Jean, rather than alienated from her as we might have been if we had been less involved in her recovery.' (Read, 1997)

Taylor (1996) also talks about 'support' or 'crisis circles':

'Over the last 20 years I have seen such circles form around a number of people. I was one of the beneficiaries of this form of ordinary human magic. People contribute to crisis support in various ways using little publicised techniques such as taking the person a meal, making them cups of tea, listening to them, letting them know someone cares and perhaps letting them scream or cry – sometimes for rather a long time, and often for much longer than a "fifty-minute hour".'

Friends can be enormously valuable to someone in distress, yet they remain largely ignored by professionals. It is also worth noting that, in most such support arrangements, many of those providing the support experience mental health problems themselves. The role that people with mental health problems can have in supporting others with similar difficulties can be critical (Chamberlin, 1977; Deegan, 1993). We have met many people with serious mental health problems who have provided support and help to their partners and friends both during mental health crises and on an ongoing basis. These include one man, seriously disabled by such difficulties, who nursed his girlfriend (who also had such problems) throughout the two years of her terminal illness in which she became progressively less able to look after herself. However, prejudices against people with mental health problems die hard. It is all too often the case that these disabled friends and partners are excluded by professionals because of their mental health problems in a way that non-disabled kin would not be.

Serious mental health problems exist in a social context and can only be understood in that context. For the individual who experiences such difficulties it is important to consider all facets of their social world. Immediate, nuclear families may be important, but they may not be the only important people in a person's life.

It is unfortunately the case that the different facets of the disabled individual's world represent different interest groups. Parents may disagree with siblings, family may disagree with friends, parents may refuse to acknowledge a lesbian or gay partner, and all may have a different perspective from the individual with mental health problems, not to mention the professionals involved. Enormous dilemmas arise for clinicians in attempting to accede to the wishes of service users, while heeding the opinions, wishes and needs of their social networks. Nevertheless, it is critical that all facets of a person's social world are considered: all may be important to the individual, all may be lost if not actively included and supported, all may be of value in helping and supporting the person, all may be central to the individual's quality of life.

11

What constitutes success? Outcome research, service monitoring and audit

Throughout the provision of healthcare questions about cost effectiveness are increasingly being asked:

'over the last five years, the issues of clinical and cost effectiveness have captured the policy agenda in the NHS as never before. Collectively (and perhaps rather belatedly) we have recognised the most important issue facing the health service is not how it should be organised or financed, but whether the care it offers actually works.' (Walshe and Ham, 1997)

It is often asserted that, hitherto, too much emphasis has been placed on the personal experience and opinions of clinicians, and too little on

'the science of health care – results from randomised controlled trials, rigorous health services research and systematic reviews of the findings from research. In short, we have neglected the scientific foundation of what we do.' (Walshe and Ham, 1997)

Such arguments have been galvanized into a pervasive policy exhortation to practice 'evidence-based healthcare' and create an 'evidence-based healthcare system'.

Although the effectiveness of healthcare has been researched and evaluated for some time, such endeavours have typically been seen by clinicians as something done by researchers and academics, quite separate from them and their day-to-day practice. For a multitude of reasons, including intense time pressures, most clinicians never engage in research and few can honestly say that they systematically keep abreast of the research work of others to ensure that their own day-to-day clinical practice is informed by the latest findings. Instead research work enters routine practice in a more haphazard fashion via clinicians reading a few papers, word of mouth and attendance at occasional conferences and training events. Clearly, such a situation risks considerable unevenness in practice, the continuation of ineffective practices and the failure to adopt new, more efficacious, approaches.

'For all the human variability it faces and the intensely personal interactions it involves, health-care is founded on knowledge acquired through the scientific method. Yet it seems we have been remarkably lax about how we direct our search for new knowledge and how we use the knowledge so painstakingly acquired through scientific enquiry.' (Walshe and Ham, 1997)

It was in response to problems such as these that the more general policy demands upon *all* clinicians to adopt evidence-based practice were directed: policies whose UK origins can be traced back to the first NHS Research and Development Strategy (DoH, 1993c). Such evidence-based healthcare involves three essential processes (Walshe and Ham, 1997):

• Evaluating the effectiveness of interventions through a rigorous programme of research conducted to high scientific standards.
• Effective distribution of the results of these evaluations in a useable form to the individuals and organizations who need them.
• Using the results of these evaluations to change clinical practice.

At first sight, such an approach seems eminently sensible. Anyone using healthcare services might reasonably expect that the treatments and interventions which they are offered are known to be effective. However, the situation is in reality far more complex than this, especially in the area of services for people with mental health problems who have multiple needs (Ridgeway, 1988; Ruggeri, 1994; Freemantle and Maynard, 1994; Bond, 1994; Blankertz, 1994; Repper and Brooker, 1998). As Mendel (1986) says:

'The difficulties of conducting outcome research are monumental and, up to present, have not been solved.'

What constitutes success: defining goals and outcomes

Any scientific or research endeavour involves a great many value judgements. In considering the effectiveness of a service or intervention, probably the most central of these judgements is what does 'effectiveness' mean? What constitutes 'success'? Such questions arise in all areas, from outcome research relating to specific treatments or interventions, through the evaluation of service systems, to the routine clinical auditing of particular facets of service performance. Too often it is assumed that symptom reduction takes pride of place and that if this can be assured everything else will follow and quality of life will necessarily be improved. This may not be the case.

'the assumption that symptom relief, reduction in the frequency of episodes of illness and improvement in functional adaptation… mean that quality of life has been enhanced may at times be unwarranted. Indeed, for some patients, these seemingly positive changes may not be accompanied by the development of meaningful interpersonal relationships, by employment that they are enthusiastic about, or by a subjective sense of satisfaction and well-being. Emphasis should be placed not only on level of clinical symptomatology or pathologic behaviour, but also on the functional integration of the patient into his or her occupational, social and cultural milieu.' (Mirin and Namerow, 1991)

These authors, like others, argue that goals of mental health services must be multi-dimensional. However, the achievement of one goal may eliminate the chances of meeting others (Dickey and Wagenaar, 1994). For example, the goals of choice and control over problems and services offered are frequently espoused by service users (Bond, 1994; Read and Reynolds, 1996) but these are incompatible with compulsory hospitalization and medication which might minimize clinical symptoms. Choices have to be made concerning definitions of success and once again, power relationships come into play (Tyrer *et al.*, 1994). The outcomes of mental health services are of interest to a great many different parties: clinicians, managers of health services, purchasers of healthcare, politicians, families, individuals and organizations in local communities, academics and researchers, not to mention service users and service user/survivor groups. As we have already discussed *'different stakeholder groups vary in their opinions about what the important outcomes are'* (Bond, 1994).

Mental health services are typically interested in such outcomes as activity figures, admission and discharge rates, use of hospital beds, the number of people living in different kinds of accommodation and so forth: those statistics which they are required to report to purchasing authorities in order to secure continued funding. Politicians and local citizens are concerned with the cost of mental healthcare as well as the rates of murder and violent crime and limiting the perceived danger and disruption to local communities. The primary interest of families is in receiving information, having their role as primary carers recognized, and receiving the support and services they need to sustain this role (Shepherd *et al.*, 1994, 1995).

Divergence in the desired goals of mental health services for all interest groups inevitably results in power struggles. For example, a provider service may demonstrate that a particular service/approach – say, intensive outreach support at home – enabled a larger number of people to live outside an institutional setting and reduced the need for hospital beds. At the same time local citizens and media may evaluate the number of beds 'lost' and protest at the closure of wards and hospitals, not to mention the increase in danger they believe to have resulted to their communities.

For the former group a decrease in beds is desirable, for the latter an increase would be preferable. Even when the outcome considered – the number of hospital beds – is the same, different value is attached to changes in different directions. Similar situations may arise in numerous areas. For example, service users may desire greater choice and options to drug treatments (Read and Reynolds, 1996), and regard as 'success' fewer people taking medication. Clinicians may regard compliance as the key issue and value positively those interventions which increase the number of people taking medication (Kemp *et al.*, 1996).

As in most areas, probably the greatest day-to-day discrepancy in the definition of goals and outcomes arises between clinicians and service users, and it is these differences that pose the greatest dilemmas for clinicians in evaluating the effectiveness of their services. Professionals typically define their primary goals in terms of reducing service users' symptoms or the frequency, duration and severity of relapses (Repper and Brooker, 1998). While service users may also desire freedom from debilitating symptoms, they typically place at least as much emphasis on the importance of decent lives:

'safe, pleasant and affordable housing, well paying and fulfilling jobs, friends... to be treated with dignity and respect, to have control over their lives and to have genuine choices. They want to feel good about themselves and to have the opportunity to achieve the same things that all of us do.' (Bond, 1994)

Numerous studies have shown differences in the goals of clinicians and service users. Dimsdale *et al.* (1979) showed that staff in a Massachusetts psychiatric unit viewed 'insight' on the part of patients as the primary goal (a view shared by Kemp *et al.*, 1996), while users themselves placed 'insight' at the bottom of their list of goals selected from a 'goal profile'. Mitchell *et al.* (1983) compared the problems listed by psychiatric patients and their physicians and found extremely low agreement even though clinicians had access to the patients' lists before making their own. Lynch and Kruzich (1986), as part of their comparison of user and professional perceptions of barriers to using mental health services, found large differences. While users identified lack of transportation and non-availability of services as the main problems, professionals translated the difficulties into psychological terms and instead blamed 'client resistance'.

More recently, despite finding some measure of agreement between service users and professionals, Shepherd *et al.* (1995) did find different priorities. Users valued help to come to terms with their problems and assistance with housing, finance, social networks and physical health, while professionals placed greater emphasis on professional support, treatment and monitoring. If professionals are pre-occupied with decreasing symptoms and time spent in hospital this may be at odds with service users' wishes for increased control and choice, and their wishes to gain employment or develop meaningful friendships (Repper and Brooker, 1998; Mirin and Namerow, 1991).

Finally, in any consideration of effectiveness, the degree to which an intervention is acceptable to service users cannot be ignored. This is particularly true for those with serious, ongoing problems who may require help, treatment and support for long periods of time, if not indefinitely, and for whom the absence of support can mean failure to survive in the community. Too often outcome trials consider only those who accepted the intervention. There are many psychiatric interventions (like ECT) that are relatively unacceptable to those who may use them and the 'drop out' rate of many services has been estimated to be around 40% (Repper and Perkins, 1995; Gournay and Brooking, 1993; Carter, 1979). In considering the effectiveness of any intervention, attention must be paid to accurate measurement of rates of 'drop out' or refusal: an intervention must be deemed ineffective if people find it so unacceptable they choose not to take it.

Measuring outcomes

Closely allied with difficulties relating to what constitutes success are a whole series of questions relating to how goals might be measured. Traditionally, concerns in this area have revolved around psychometric properties: the reliability, validity and sensitivity of the assessment measures employed (Guildford, 1954; Cronbach, 1971). While these are clearly important there are many other issues that require consideration. As Bachrach (1982) suggests:

'If effective outcome research is to be performed, it is necessary not only to state program goals with exactness but also to use measures that reflect progress in the attainment of those particular goals.'

The selection of appropriate measures clearly involves a greater degree of precision in the specification of goals than is common in most mental health services. For example, simply in relation to symptoms there may be numerous goals: to reduce the actual symptoms that the person displays; to reduce the distress they experience; to reduce the extent to which they are prevented from engaging in other desired activities; to change the behaviour associated with their symptoms; to enable a person to gain a greater sense of control over their symptoms and so forth. Clearly, each of these requires different assessment instruments. It is not sufficient to assume that a set of factors such as these co-vary. Strauss (1994) argued that people who do not demonstrate a marked improvement in symptoms or social functioning – those things which outcome studies typically address – may still report an increased sense of control or increased understanding of their problems which might reduce their feelings of hopelessness and distress. There is, for example, no necessary connection between a reduction in the severity of a person's symptoms and their sense of control or engagement in other activities: any such correlations are essentially empirical questions that must be tested.

Services for people who experience serious ongoing mental health problems typically have multiple goals and therefore require multiple outcome measures. Given the differences between the goals of different stakeholders, it would seem important to have different outcome measures reflecting the interests of these stakeholders. To some extent this does happen. Those concerned about public safety collect data on the number of murders (and other crimes) committed by people with mental health problems. However, few if any powerful interest groups are interested in the positive contribution that people with mental health problems make to communities, so little data is collected in this area. Those who have an eye on the public purse collect data on bed usage and the amount of money going into mental hospitals. However, most outcome measures have been devised by clinicians working within services. Those who provide the treatment also devise the ways to tell if that treatment has worked – not exactly an independent evaluation! The one important interest group which has not hitherto been involved in devising measures to evaluate the outcome of the services they receive are service users themselves. This shortcoming matters.

If outcome measures are all designed by clinicians then they will reflect clinicians' agendas and concerns. This is apparent in the numerous instruments for measuring symptoms and social functioning, and the almost complete absence of tools for measuring the choice, control and personal fulfilment that service users value. Even the large number of 'patient satisfaction' scales available have been devised by clinicians (Ruggeri, 1994). The one notable exception to this is a consumer-constructed scale to measure empowerment among users of mental health services (Rogers *et al.*, 1997). As many services claim to want to 'empower' their users, the authors developed a scale to measure this construct. Adopting principles of participatory action research (Rogers and Palmer-Erbs, 1994) a board of 10 leading members of the user/survivor movement in the USA (reflecting the diversities within that movement) was convened by one of the user researchers. This board began by developing a definition of the attributes of empowerment for people with mental health problems (Rogers *et al.*, 1997). These included:

- having decision-making power
- having access to information and resources
- having a range of options from which to take choices (not just yes–no and either–or)
- a feeling that one can make a difference (being hopeful)
- learning to think critically, unlearning conditioning and seeing things differently. For example, learning to redefine who one is (speaking in one's own voice), learning to redefine what one can do, and learning to redefine one's relationships with institutionalized power
- learning about and expressing anger

- not feeling alone and feeling part of a group
- understanding that a person has rights
- effecting change in one's life and community
- learning skills, e.g. communication, that one defines as important
- changing others' perceptions of one's competency and capacity to act
- coming out of the closet
- growth and change that is never-ending and self-initiated
- increasing one's positive self-image and overcoming stigma.

Using these attributes of empowerment, a scale was developed and tested. Good psychometric properties (internal consistency, construct validity, known groups validity) were demonstrated and a factor analysis revealed five factors:

1 self-esteem and self-efficacy
2 power and powerlessness
3 community activism and autonomy
4 optimism and control over the future
5 righteous anger.

The final scale therefore offers a way of evaluating the extent to which services are achieving the user-defined goal of empowerment.

While this scale adopted some more innovative research models derived from participatory action research, its product was a traditional questionnaire. Other methodologies might also be helpful in enabling evaluations to be conducted on the basis of a service user agenda. For example, focus groups can be used to good effect (Repper *et al.*, 1998; Kitzinger, 1995) allowing service users to develop their thoughts and ideas with each other and minimizing the extent to which a professionally set agenda is imposed. Steele (1992) has suggested a number of formal and informal methods via which consumer appraisal might be used to evaluate services. These include diaries kept by users and 'user-councils' – standing groups of users who are regularly involved and consulted.

However, it is not simply in the area of the design of outcome measures that important methodological questions arise, there are also issues relating to their administration. It has long been recognized that if clinicians complete outcome measures on their own interventions and services then biases can creep in: professionals understandably wish to portray their work in a positive light. However, the simple use of an independent staff researcher does not resolve all difficulties. The person often continues to be construed as a staff member by service users who understandably (and despite protestations to the contrary) may have no reason to trust that the care they receive will not be influenced by their answers. Srebnick *et al.* (1990) described how, in assessments of consumer preference and satisfaction, an acquiescent response set can be induced: service users endeavour to please the questioner by saying what they wish them to hear. They go on to suggest that one way to avoid this is to involve service users as researchers. Service users trained to perform assessments and interviews are more likely to be able to offer proper reassurance to those whom they interview and obtain richer, more accurate information about their problems and concerns.

The heterogeneous nature of the population and their difficulties

A further dilemma in evaluating interventions and services comes from the extremely heterogeneous nature of the people who have mental health problems. From a research and evaluation perspective such differences are important as the same intervention or service is unlikely to serve all people equally well. Numerous demographic distinctions exist in terms of age, class, gender, disability, lesbian/gay and race/ethnicity: there is evidence that services may not provide well for people from some minority racial/ethnic groups (Frederick, 1991) or women (Repper *et al.*, 1998). From a professional perspective distinctions between people are typically made in clinical terms – however it is important to remember that these interact with such demographic variables and so a 60-year old Asian woman with a diagnosis of schizophrenia is not the same as a 20-year old African Caribbean man with the same diagnosis, and they will need different treatments and services.

Diagnosis is, of course, a major way of defining clinical subgroups, but in addition some behavioural and service usage characteristics may be employed: duration of service contact, level of disability, safety (both public and individual) and support (DoH, 1995a). Even at the apparently simple level of diagnosis, there are many difficulties. The population with serious mental health problems is made up of people with a great range of diagnoses, from the most common – schizophrenia – through affective, organic and anxiety-based difficulties to a range of 'personality disorders'. Yet the literature seems to have assumed that interventions and services for those with a diagnosis of schizophrenia can be applied to the larger population of all those who have serious and ongoing mental health problems (Repper and Brooker, 1998). There is, however, no empirical evidence that this is the case: any evaluation of a treatment, intervention or service must explore the relative effectiveness for people with different diagnoses. While it may be possible to gain separate information for the more numerous diagnostic groups, it may be difficult to do so for less numerous ones. Consequently, in working in a long-term care setting with people who experience Korsakoff's psychosis, or who are seriously disabled and have a diagnosis of personality disorder, the clinician is often left guessing whether, for example, family interventions will work, or whether sheltered work will be beneficial.

To add to these dilemmas are the problems of multiple diagnoses. There may have been a set of interventions developed for people with a diagnosis of schizophrenia, but are these equally effective for someone with such a diagnosis who also has learning difficulties and pre-lingual deafness? In addition, there is considerable evidence of the great range of difficulties which people manifest within a single diagnostic entity. Schizophrenia is the most often cited in this regard (*see* Boyle, 1990; Bentall, 1990) with its myriad different courses and symptom patterns. So when a particular intervention is effective for someone who experiences passivity pheno-mena relatively continually, is it equally effective for someone who experiences such ideas only episodically? Is it equally effective for someone who experiences no such ideas but is troubled by hearing voices? Does it help someone who is particularly distressed by their symptoms as much as someone who is not so distressed?

It is not only clinicians who make distinctions between different groups of service users. Users also recognize distinctions within their own numbers. For example, those involved in the user movement and those who are not, and within this group, anti-psychiatry 'survivors' and more reformist 'users'. The range of differences is well illus-trated in the diverse set of contributions collected by Read and Reynolds (1996): some valued medication and ECT while others did not, some reported positive encounters with in-patient settings and professionals while others wanted real alternatives out-side mainstream services. From a research perspective, the purpose of making distinc-tions between different groups of service users is to facilitate investigation of their different needs and the differential effectiveness of alternative types of service provi-sion. It is likely to be important to move beyond simple diagnostic distinctions to in-vestigate more effective ways of providing services to people of different ages, races and cultures and to people with different beliefs and attitudes about mental health issues.

The heterogeneous nature of interventions and their interactions

In any mental health context it is extremely difficult to evaluate the effectiveness of a single intervention in isolation from others. As Mendel (1986) argued:

'The problem of defining treatment and identifying the specific variables which represent the significant interventions is complex.'

It is usually impossible to alter variables singly in order to evaluate the relative con-tribution of different components, or even to define all the variables introduced in treatment interventions (Meltzoff and Kornreich, 1970). Even in relatively simple psychopharmacological research it is hard to evaluate the effect of the psychological component of medicine administration, the importance of hope and positive expect-ancy on the part of the user and the physician's view of the medication (Luborsky *et al.*, 1971, 1983).

'There is much evidence to show that the effectiveness of a particular medication in the hands of one physician is statistically significantly different from the effectiveness of the same

medication in the hands of another, the difference being the personality of the physicians and the ability of the therapists to form therapeutic alliances with their patients in producing a hopeful expectancy.' (Mendel, 1986)

Services for people who have serious mental health problems rarely comprise the administration of a single drug or treatment. The multiple problems and needs of a diverse population of users dictate that services are multi-faceted, and therefore the difficulties are magnified. It is often quite difficult to describe all the components of services which may cut across agencies in the statutory, voluntary and private sectors. With a few exceptions (e.g. Hogarty *et al.*, 1986, where three components were examined) studies typically examine one particular facet of intervention (e.g. coping skills enhancement as a specific strategy for managing hallucinations and delusions) and ignore all other aspects of intervention including the possible interactions between these and the target intervention. All that such studies really examine is the incremental effect of introducing a particular element to an already complex service.

Alternatively, studies have reduced a complex set of components to a single umbrella intervention. For example, there have been studies of care management (Ford *et al.*, 1995) in which the term 'care management' is used to cover a complex set of multiple interventions. While there may be some commonalities across people (like a written care plan, standard assessments performed etc.) everything else may vary so that no two individuals are receiving the same interventions, help and support although all are getting 'care management'. Such studies really contribute little except to say whether a complex (but unspecified) array of services 'works' according to certain criteria. It does not allow the key components, or the relationship between particular components and particular outcomes, to be identified. It thus makes it hard for the approach to be transferred to different settings: it would be hard to contemplate the precise replication of the full range of statutory and voluntary services available together with the ordinary resources available in the community where the study was performed. For example, a measured increase in satisfaction or quality of life may have nothing to do with regular visits from a key-worker, but rather to the presence of a bingo hall or dog track to which the key-worker was able to take the person. Attributing particular changes to specific interventions can be extremely difficult.

Designing evaluations

There are numerous possible approaches to describing and evaluating services: from the tightly controlled outcome trial with randomization of carefully matched patients into specific, well-defined, treatment subgroups, through more naturalistic observation of the effects of a particular intervention on a wide range of people in an ordinary service setting and evaluations of the outcomes of whole service systems, to audits of specific aspects of services. The most appropriate designs for evaluations undoubtedly depend upon the questions being asked.

A purchaser of healthcare may well ask whether a service 'works' on some criteria. If so, simply taking 'before' and 'after' measures on that criterion may suffice. However, such an approach cannot answer questions about whether doing nothing, or doing something else, would have worked equally well. It cannot determine which element of the service produced any positive results or why. If no changes are found it is impossible to tell whether this means that the service was ineffective or whether it was, in fact, successfully preventing deterioration and effectively maintaining the status quo. These latter possibilities are particularly important in the context of services for people who experience serious ongoing disabilities: the absence of change – preventing deterioration and maintaining a person's quality of life and functioning – may be critical.

In order to answer questions about whether one approach is 'better' than another on some criterion variable, comparison groups are necessary. This can often most practically be achieved by comparing people in two or more existing services. While this can provide more information than a simple before/after design, questions can still be raised about whether the differences found might be due to differences between the people using or referred to the different services, or to extraneous differences between the services and their circumstances.

In order to resolve some of these difficulties, the random allocation to groups has been used as a way of trying to ensure that any differences found are a consequence of the intervention and not of existing inter-group differences. Much of the pioneering work on the effectiveness of community care for people who experience serious mental health problems involved the random allocation of people to one of two complete programmes (Stein and Test, 1980), e.g. an assertive community treatment group and a standard outpatient follow-up group. While such studies generate greater confidence that any differences found resulted from some aspect of the particular programmes considered, the multi-faceted nature of the programmes prevented the precise reasons for such differences from being ascertained. For example, in an assertive outreach programme, it may be regular visits from a key-worker, a supportive relationship with a key-worker, help to get money, help to get and keep a job, help with relationships, help to adjust to and live with disabilities, help to take medication, help available 24 hours a day in crisis, the possibility of respite admissions or any complex interaction of these that is effective. Further, it may be something about user and clinician expectations that is critical, especially as such trials invariably involve a comparison between something new and something that has gone before. Users know that they are receiving something new and different and therefore may have positive expectations, and the belief that one can do things increases the likelihood of success. Similarly, clinicians have been recruited to a new and exciting project and have an investment in making it 'work' in a way that those practising with established methods may not have.

In order to begin attributing changes to specific interventions, greater precision and a tighter experimental design are needed to examine the effects of specific variables, e.g. the effect of a particular treatment rather than the effect of expectations. The double-blind, randomized controlled trial has always been seen as the gold standard of clinical outcome research. That is, the random allocation of a clearly identified group of people to one or more different specific interventions in such a way that neither user, clinician or researcher is aware of which group each person is in. This means that differences between groups might confidently be said to reflect differences in the effectiveness of treatments. However, even in its traditional 'home land' – the evaluation of new drugs – such randomized controlled trials have been severely criticized (Freemantle and Maynard, 1994). Gotzshe (1989) has listed some 22 factors that may artificially increase the number and the proportion of significant results favouring a new drug. These include selection of patients dissatisfied with a control drug, choice of dose, selective reporting among many variables, ineffective blinding, handling of withdrawals, uneven distribution of prognostic factors, sub-group analyses, selective reporting of significance levels and publication bias.

Unfortunately, double-blind, randomized controlled trials are rarely useful in assessing the outcomes of interventions and services for people with serious mental health problems. The aim of random allocation to groups is to ensure the absence of systematic differences between groups on variables other than the intervention being tested. We have already discussed the difficulties arising from the diversity of the population and their problems, and the ways in which sub-groups might be defined, together with those resulting from heterogeneous and interactive interventions. It may be possible in a few instances to randomly allocate individuals to a particular treatment (or not) while keeping all other service variables constant (care management, emergency services, day services, key-worker systems etc.). However, this does not strictly test the effect of the particular treatment, rather it tests the incremental effect of the treatment in combination with the other services. It is not, therefore, possible to conclude that the intervention is effective, rather that it is effective in conjunction with these other elements.

A technique used in some areas of mental health research is the no-treatment – 'waiting list' – control group: comparing the progress of those on the waiting list with those receiving a specific intervention. Where people have multiple and pressing needs as in the case of those with serious mental health problems, such a 'no-treatment' condition is rarely possible. Instead, the individual generally receives support from another service (acute ward, voluntary sector etc.) while waiting which, from an experimental point of view, is quite a different thing.

At the other end of the scale, issues of when interventions 'finish' can confound researchers. Where mental health interventions are brief and time-limited, or where they are expected to have their desired effect over a short period, it is clear when the effects might be measured. Even still there is a balance between short follow-up, which allows the effects of intervention to be evaluated but not their durability across time, and longer follow-up which measures durability across time but may be confounded by other variables and events unrelated to the initial intervention. When a person has ongoing mental health problems the situation can be even more complex. While clinicians may focus on symptom control which may reasonably be expected in a relatively short time frame, many users focus on more general issues about their lives. As many have argued, the process of recovery is long, if not life-long (Deegan, 1988, 1990, 1992, 1993; Anthony, 1994). Interventions which might facilitate a person's recovery and rebuilding their life in the longer term may in the short term appear ineffective and be abandoned in favour of those which may have shorter-term benefits but lack longer-term effectiveness.

Finally, there is the issue of whether clinicians and service users can be 'blind' to which group they are in. Even in the arena of drugs, it is somewhat naive to assume that people, who may have taken many different types of medication, are honestly unaware whether what they are taking now is something new or something they have taken before. Most people report feeling different (for good or bad) when their medication is changed. However, when one moves beyond pills, the idea of anyone being 'blind' to which intervention is which is ludicrous. Behaviour therapy and analytic psychotherapy look and feel quite different and it is impossible not to notice that someone has called at your house three times in the last week if you are in the 'intensive outreach' condition. Psychosocial (and probably psychopharmacological) interventions will always be confounded by the beliefs and expectations of those who use them and those who administer them.

When we do not know

Despite the many problems that arise in evaluating success of services it is undoubtedly the case that clinicians have to answer the questions of both service users and purchasers about what their interventions and services do. In order to answer such questions the initial issue is again an ethical or political one: what does 'working' mean? Different interest groups have different views that will lead to different interventions being considered effective. If the outcome which is valued is the recipient feeling good then massage or aromatherapy may rate highly. If the valued outcome is diminution of active psychotic symptoms then neuroleptics might be preferred. If the valued outcome is public safety then locked facilities and compulsory treatment might fare highly. If the valued outcome is enabling users to get a job then supported employment may be the intervention of choice. Different interventions are undoubtedly better at achieving different ends with different people and such differences should be reflected in outcome research and service evaluation.

Just as there will never be a single intervention to address all the needs of someone who is seriously disabled by mental health problems, so there will never be a single definitive experiment which proves which intervention is best. But this does not mean that research is unimportant. Rather, the process of research, evaluation and audit must be seen as incremental with every clinician asking questions about what they do and answering them either by reference to information they can collect as part of their work, or via the information collected and published by others. Even when an intervention is known to be generally effective, there is not a single approach or treatment that has proved effective with everyone. Each individual brings a different set of problems, preferences, beliefs, assets and skills. Therefore, at the bottom line, we need to adopt an 'experimental' method with each individual (Kazdin, 1982). Working together with the service user to decide what they want to achieve and how best to achieve it, trying it, evaluating the extent to which their goals are achieved, and rethinking when things have not turned out as planned.

Increasingly the process of research and evaluation, at the level of individuals, services and interventions, must include those people who are the recipients of these ministrations as experts in both the nature of the problems they experience and the effects (and effectiveness) of different interventions and approaches. As Srebnick *et al.* (1990) argued:

'Traditional research methods have emphasised designs which presume the centrality of intervention by professionals, rather than the phenomenology and personal experience of consumers themselves. These strategies tend to objectify human experience and create distance between the researcher and informant.'

It is not particularly illuminating simply to ask general questions about 'user satisfaction' with services as defined by clinician-constructed rating scales:

'... most studies on satisfaction with health care and mental health services show that the majority of respondents are satisfied (approximately 75%).' (Ruggeri, 1994)

It is necessary to give service users greater power in the whole proceedings to define what they consider to be the relevant goals and how these might best be measured. It would be very informative to examine the different interventions and treatments currently on offer in terms of their success in achieving user-defined, as well as clinician-defined, desirable outcomes. Data already exists about what service users want from services, perhaps it is now time to start evaluating services in these terms.

References

Aday LA and Andersen R (1974) A framework for the study of access to medical care. *Health Services Research*. **9**: 208–20.

Anciano D and Kirkpatrick A (1990) CMHTs and clinical psychology: the death of a profession? *Clinical Psychology Forum*. **April**: 9-12.

Anthony LA (1977) Psychological rehabilitation: a concept of need in a method. *American Psychologist*. **August**: 658–62.

Anthony WA (1994) Recovery from mental illness: the guiding vision of the mental health system in the 1990s. In: The Publication Committee of IASPRS (ed) *An Introduction to Psychiatric Rehabilitation*. International Association of Psychosocial Rehabilitation Services, Columbia, MD.

Antonovsky A and Hartmann H (1974) Delay in the detection of cancer: a review of the literature. *Health Education Monographs*. **2**: 98–125.

Atkinson JM (1991) Autonomy and mental health. In: P Barker and S Baldwin (eds) *Ethical Issues in Mental Health*. Chapman and Hall, London.

Atkinson JM and Coia DA (1989) Reponsibility to carers: an ethical dilemma. *Psychiatric Bulletin*. **13**: 603–4.

Atkinson JM and Coia DA (1995) *Families Coping with Schizophrenia: a practitioner's guide to family groups*. John Wiley and Sons, Chichester.

Atkisson C (1992) Clinical services research: Report of the clinical services research panel, National Institute of Mental Health. *Schizophrenia Bulletin*. **18**: 561–626.

American Psychological Association (1993) *Guidelines for Non-handicapping Language*. American Psychological Association, Washington DC.

Ananth J (1984) Physical illness and psychiatric disorders. *Comprehensive Psychiatry*. **25**: 595.

Awad AG (1993) Subjective response to neuroleptics in schizophrenia. *Schizophrenia Bulletin*. **19**: 609–16.

Babiker IE (1986) Non-compliance in schizophrenia. *Psychiatric Developments.* **4**: 329–37.

Bachrach LL (1982) Assessment of outcomes in community support systems: results, problems and limitations. *Hospital and Community Psychiatry.* **8**: 39–61.

Bachrach LL (1988a) Defining mental illness: a concept paper. *Hospital and Community Psychiatry.* **40**: 234–5.

Bachrach LL (1988b) Community mental health centres and other semantic concerns. *Hospital and Community Psychiatry.* **39**: 605–6.

Bachrach LL (1989) The legacy of model programmes. *Hospital and Community Psychiatry.* **40**: 234–45.

Baker P (1995) *The Voice Inside: a practical guide to coping with hearing voices.* Hearing Voices Network, Manchester.

Barker P (1997) In: Book Reviews. *Journal of Mental Health and Psychiatric Nursing.* **4**: 316–17.

Barker I and Peck E (1996) User empowerment: a decade of experience. *The Mental Health Review.* **1**: 5–13.

Barnes M (1996) Introducing the issues. In: R Perkins, Z Nadirshaw, J Copperman *et al.* (eds) *Women in Context: good practices in mental health services for women.* GPMH, London.

Bateson G, Jackson DD and Haley J (1956) Towards a theory of schizophrenia. *Behavioural Science.* **1**: 251–64.

Bean J, Keller C, Newburg C *et al.* (1989) Methods for the reduction of AIDS social anxiety and social stigma. *AIDS Education and Prevention.* **1**: 194–221.

Becker MH (1974) The health belief model and personal health behaviour. *Health Education Monograph.* **2**(4): 324–508.

Becker MH and Rosenstock IM (1984) Compliance with medical advice. In: MH Becker and IM Rosenstock (eds) *Health Care and Human Behaviour.* Academic Press, London.

Becker MH, Radius SM, Rosenstock IM *et al.* (1978) Compliance with a medical regimen for asthma: a test of the health belief model. *Public Health Reports.* **93**: 268–77.

Beeforth M, Conlan E and Graley R (1994) *Have We Got Views For You? User Evaluation of Case Management.* Sainsbury Centre for Mental Health, London.

Beeforth M, Conlan E, Field V *et al.* (1990) *Whose Service Is It Anyway?* Sainsbury Centre for Mental Health, London.

Bentall RP (ed) (1990) *Reconstructing Schizophrenia.* Routledge, London.

Bentall RP, Jackson HF and Pilgrim D (1988) Abandoning the concept of 'schizophrenia': some implications of validity arguments for psychological research into psychotic phenomena. *British Journal of Clinical Psychology.* **27**: 156–9.

Besio SW, Blach AK and Quinn K (1987) *The Role of Ex-Patients and Consumers in Human Resource Development for the 1990's.* Center for Community Change through Housing and Support, Burlington, VT.

Bingley W (1990) *An Introduction to Advocacy*. Good Practices in Mental Health Information Pack, London.

Birchwood M (1998) Early intervention in psychotic relapse. In: C Brooker and J Repper (eds) *Policy, Practice and Research in Community Mental Health Services*. Bailliere Tindall, London.

Birchwood M and Shepherd G (1992) Controversies and growing points in cognitive behavioural interventions for people with schizophrenia. *Behavioural Psychotherapy*. **20**: 305–42.

Birchwood M, Hallett S and Preston M (1988) *Schizophrenia: an integrated approach to research treatment*. Longman, Harlow.

Birchwood M, Cochrane R, Macmillan JF *et al.* (1992) The influence of ethnicity and family structure on relapse in first episode schizophrenia. *British Journal of Psychiatry*. **161**: 783–90.

Birley J (1991) Schizophrenia: the problems of handicap. In: D Bennett and H Freeman (eds) *Community Psychiatry*. Churchill Livingstone, London.

Blackwell B (1972) The drug defaulter. *Clinical Pharmacology and Therapeutics*. **13**: 841–8.

Blanch AK (1991) Issue paper: stigma and discrimination in mental health. *Community Support Network News*. **No. 2**.

Blankertz L (1994) Evaluating psychiatric rehabilitation programmes. In: The Publication Committee of IASPRS (ed) *An Introduction to Psychiatric Rehabilitation*. International Association of Psychosocial Rehabilitation Services, Columbia, MD.

Bond GR (1994) Psychiatric rehabilitation outcome. In: The Publication Committee of IASPRS (ed) *An Introduction to Psychiatric Rehabilitation*. International Association of Psychosocial Rehabilitation Services, Columbia, MD.

Bond GR, Drake RE, Mueser KT *et al.* (1997) An update on supported employment for people with severe mental illness. *Psychiatric Services*. **48**: 335–46.

Bonhoustos J, Holroyd J, Leman H *et al.* (1983) Sexual intimacies between psychotherapists and patients. *Professional Research and Practice*. **14**(2): 185–96.

Bord R (1971) Rejection of the mentally ill: continuities and further developments. *Social Problems*. **18**(4): 496–509.

Bowl R (1996) Involving service users in mental health services: social services departments and the NHS and Community Care Act 1990. *Journal of Mental Health*. **5**: 287–303.

Boyle M (1990) *Scizophrenia: a scientific delusion?* Routledge, London.

Brandon D (1991) User power. In: P Barker and S Baldwin (eds) *Ethical Issues in Mental Health*. Chapman and Hall, London.

Breeze J and Repper J (1998) Struggling for control: the care experiences of difficult patients in mental health services. Accepted for publication by *Journal of Advanced Nursing*.

Brewin C, Wing JK and Mangen S (1987) Principles and practice of measuring needs in the long term mentally ill: the MRC Needs For Care Assessment. *Psychological Medicine*. **17**: 971–81.

Brewin C, Wing JK and Mangen S (1988) Needs for care among long term mentally ill: report from the Camberwell High Contact Survey. *Psychological Medicine*. **18**: 457–68.

Briere J and Runtz M (1987) Post-sexual abuse trauma: data and implications for clinical practice. *Journal of Interpersonal Violence*. **1**: 367–79.

British Psychological Society (1992) The core purpose and philosophy of the profession. *Clinical Psychology Forum*. **April**: 34–6.

Brooker C and Conway P (1995) *A Census of Clients on CPN Caseloads in Community Health Sheffield*. Sheffield Centre for Health and Related Research, Sheffield.

Brooker C, Repper J and Booth A (1996) The effectiveness of community mental health nursing: a review. *Journal of Clinical Effectiveness*. **1**: 1–7.

Brown GW and Birley JLT (1968) Crises and life changes and the onset of schizophrenia. *Journal of Health and Social Behaviour*. **9**: 203–14.

Brown GW and Harris T (1978) *The Social Origins of Depression*. Tavistock, London.

Brown GW and Rutter LM (1966) The measurement of family activities and relationships. *Human Relations*. **19**: 241–63.

Brown GW, Carstairs GM and Topping GC (1958) The post-hospital adjustment of chronic mental patients. *Lancet*. **ii**: 685–9.

Brown GW, Birley JLT and Wing JK (1972) Influence of family life on the course of schizophrenic disorders: a replication. *British Journal of Psychiatry*. **121**: 241–58.

Bryant L and McClelland F (1997) *Advance Directives: making them work for people who have mental health problems*. Paper given at MIND Annual Conference, Scarborough, November 1997.

Buchanon RW (1995) Clozapine. *Schizophrenia Bulletin*. **21**: 579–92.

Bynoe I (1993) New targets for a magic bullet. *Care in the Community*. **February**: 4–5.

Campbell P (1996a) Challenging loss of power. In: J Read and J Reynolds (eds) *Speaking Our Minds*. Open University Press, Milton Keynes.

Campbell P (1996b) User action: the last ten years. *The Mental Health Review*. **1**(4): 14–15.

Campbell P (1996c) What users want from mental health crisis services. *The Mental Health Review*. **1**(1): 19–21.

Campbell P (1997) Citizen Smith. *Nursing Times*. **93**: 31–2.

Campbell D and Draper R (1985) *Applications of Systemic Family Therapy*. Grune and Stratton, London.

Carter J (1979) *Somewhere to Go: about Adult Day Centres*. National Institute of Social Work, London.

Carling P (1994) *Language: a tool for change*. CMHA Waterloo Regional Branch, Ontario.

Carvel J (1991) Therapy scheme for rapists. *Guardian*. **May 21**: 3.

Chamberlin J (1977) *On Our Own*. McGraw Hill, New York.

Chamberlin J (1984) Speaking for ourselves: an overview of the ex-psychiatric inmates movement. *Psychosocial Rehabilitation Journal*. **515**: 3–11.

Chamberlin J (1990) The ex-patients' movement: where we've been and where we're going. *Journal of Mind and Behaviour*. **11**(3/4): 324–36.

Clifford P, Craig T and Sayce L (1988) *Towards Co-ordinated Care for People with Long-term Severe Mental Illness*. Sainsbury Centre for Mental Health, London.

Clinical Standards Advisory Group (1995) *Schizophrenia. Volume 1*. HMSO, London.

Conrad P (1985) The meaning of medications: another look at compliance. *Social Science and Medicine*. **20**: 29-37.

Cook JA and Pickett SA (1987) Feelings of burden and criticalness among parents residing with chronically mentally ill offspring. *Journal of Applied Social Science*. **12**: 79-107.

Conlan E (1996) Shaking hands with the devil. In: J Read and J Reynolds (eds) *Speaking Our Minds*. Open University Press, Milton Keynes.

Conlan E, Gell C, Graley R *et al.* (1994) *User Group Advocacy: a code of practice*. Mental Health Task Force, Department of Health, London.

Conning A and Rowland LA (1992) Staff attitudes and the provision of individualised care: what determines what people do for people with long term psychiatric disabilities? *Journal of Mental Health*. **1**: 78–80.

Corrigan PW, Liberman RP and Fugel JD (1990) From neuroleptic non-compliance to collaboration in the treatment of schizophrenia. *Hospital and Community Psychiatry*. **41**: 1203–11.

Creer C, Sturt E and Wykes T (1982) The role of relatives. In: JK Wing (ed) *Long Term Community Care: experience in a London borough*. Psychological Medicine, Monograph Supplement. **2**: 29–39.

Crepaz-Keay D (1996) Who do *you* represent? In: J Read and J Reynolds (eds) *Speaking Our Minds*. Open University Press, Milton Keynes.

Cumming E and Cumming J (1957) *Closed Ranks: an experiment in mental health*. Harvard University Press, Cambridge, MA.

Crail M (1997) Dissatisfaction guaranteed. *Health Service Journal*. **16 October**: 13.

Cronbach LJ (1971) Test validation. In: RL Thorndike (ed) *Educational Measurement*. American Council for Education, Washington DC.

Daly M (1978) *Gyn/Ecology: the metaethics of radical feminism*. The Women's Press, London.

Davey B (1994) Madness and its causative contexts. *Changes*. **12**: 113–31.

David AS (1990) Insight and psychosis. *British Journal of Psychiatry*. **156**: 798–808.

Davidson B and Perkins R (1997) Mad to work here … *Nursing Times*. **93**: 27–30.

Davies N, Lingham R, Prior C *et al.* (1995) *Report of the Inquiry into the Circumstances Leading to the Death of Jonathon Newby (a volunteer worker) on 9th October 1993 in Oxford.* HMSO, London.

Davis LM and Drummond MF (1990) The economic burden of schizophrenia. *Psychiatric Bulletin.* **14**: 522–5.

Dear M and Gleeson B (1991) Community attitudes towards the homeless. *Urban Geography.* **12**(2): 155–76.

Deegan P (1988) Recovery: the lived experience of rehabilitation. *Psychosocial Rehabilitation Journal.* **11**: 11–19.

Deegan P (1990) *How Recovery Begins.* The Center for Community Change Through Housing and Support, Burlington, VT.

Deegan P (1992) *Recovery, Rehabilitation and the Conspiracy of Hope: a keynote address.* The Center for Community Change Through Housing and Support, Burlington, VT.

Deegan PE (1993) Recovering our sense of value after being labelled. *Journal of Psychosocial Nursing.* **31**: 7–11.

Diamond RJ (1983) Enhancing medication use in schizophrenic patients. *Journal of Clinical Psychiatry.* **44**: 7–14.

Dickey B and Wagenaar H (1994) Evaluating mental health care reform: including the clinician, client and family perspective. *The Journal of Mental Health Administration.* **21**: 313–19.

Dimsdale JE, Klerman G and Shershow JC (1979) Conflict in treatment goals between patients and staff. *Social Psychiatry.* **14**: 1–4.

Dixon LB and Lehman AF (1995) Family interventions for schizophrenia. *Schizophrenia Bulletin.* **21**: 631–43.

DoH (1989a) *Working for Patients.* Cmnd 555. HMSO, London.

DoH (1989b) *Caring for People.* Cmnd 849. HMSO, London.

DoH (1989c) *Community Care: agenda for action.* HMSO, London.

DoH (1990) *NHS and Community Care Act.* HMSO, London.

DoH (1991a) *Health of the Nation.* Cmnd 1523. HMSO, London.

DoH/Scottish Office (1991b) *Care Management and Assessment: managers guide.* HMSO, London.

DoH/NHS Executive (1993a) *Monitoring the Patient's Charter: good practice guide.* HMSO, London.

DoH (1993b) *Health of the Nation Key Area Handbook: mental illness.* HMSO, London.

DoH (1993c) *Research for Health.* HMSO, London.

DoH (1994a) *Guidance on the Discharge of Mentally Disordered People and Their Continuing Care in the Community.* HMSO, London.

DoH (1994b) *Introduction of Supervision Registers for Mentally Ill People with a Mental Illness Referred to Specialist Psychiatric Services*. HMSO, London.

DoH (1994c) *Working in Partnership*. HMSO, London.

DoH (1995a) *Building Bridges: a guide to arrangements for inter-agency working for the care and protection of severely mentally ill people*. HMSO, London.

DoH (1995b) *The Mental Health (Patients in the Community) Act*. HMSO, London.

DoH/ NHS Executive (1996) *Primary Care: the future*. HMSO, London.

Doll W (1976) Family coping with the mentally ill: an unanticipated problem of deinstitutionalisation. *Hospital and Community Psychiatry*. **27**: 183–5.

Donovan JE and Blake DR (1992) Patient non-compliance: deviance or reasoned decision making. *Social Science and Medicine*. **34**: 507–13.

Eckman TA, Wirshing WC, Marder SR *et al.* (1992) Technique for training patients in illness self-management: a controlled trial. *American Journal of Psychiatry*. **149**: 1549–55.

Eisen SA and Miller DK (1990) The effect of prescribed daily dose frequency on patient medication compliance. *Archives of Internal Medicine*. **150:** 1881–4.

Ekdawi M and Conning A (1994) *Psychiatric Rehabilitation: a practical guide*. Chapman and Hall, London.

Estroff S (1993) *Community Mental Health Services: extinct, endangered or evolving?* Paper presented at the *Mental Health Practices in the Nineties: changes and challenges Conference*. Silver Springs, MD.

Fadden G, Bebbington P and Kuipers L (1987) The burden of care: the impact of functional psychiatric illness on the patient's family. *British Journal of Psychiatry*. **150**: 285–92.

Falloon I, Boyd J and McGill C (1984) Family management in the prevention of exacerbations of schizophrenia: a controlled study. *New England Journal of Medicine*. **306**: 1437–40.

Fattah EA (1982) Public opposition to prison alternatives and community corrections: a strategy for action. *Canadian Journal of Criminology*. **24**(4): 371–84.

Fernando S (1991) *Mental Health, Race and Culture*. MIND/Macmillan, London.

Ferrera JA and Vizarro C (1988) *Expressed Emotion and the Course of Schizophrenia in a Spanish Sample*. Paper presented at the *19th Annual Congress of the European Association of Behavioural Therapy*. Vienna, September 20–24.

Fleischhaker WW, Meise U, Gunther V *et al.* (1994) Compliance with antipsychotic drug treatment: influence of side effects. *Acta Psychiatrica Scandanavica*. **89**(suppl 382): 11–15.

Ford R, Beadsmoore A, Ryan P *et al.* (1995) Providing the safety net: case management for people with a serious mental illness. *Journal of Mental Health*. **1**: 91–9.

Foucault M (1967) *Madness and Civilisation*. Tavistock, London.

Frank E, Kupfer DJ and Siegel LR (1995) Alliance or compliance: a philosophy of outpatient care. *Journal of Clinical Psychology.* **56**(Jan suppl): 11–17.

Frederick J (1991) *Positive Thinking for Mental Health.* Black Mental Health Group, London.

Freemantle N and Maynard A (1994) Something rotten in the state of clinical and economic evaluations? *Health Economics.* **3**: 63–7.

Fromm-Reichmann F (1948) Notes on the development of schizophrenia by psychoanalytic psychotherapy. *Psychiatry.* **11**: 262–73.

GM (zapped) (1994) A shock to the system. *Breakthrough.* **1**(1): 5.

Ganster DC and Victor B (1988) The impact of social support on mental and physical health. *British Journal of Medical Psychology.* **61**: 17.

Gardner J and Hill O (1994) Compliance with depot medication and readmission to hospital in patients with schizophrenia. *Psychiatric Bulletin.* **18**: 660–1.

Garrity TF (1981) Medical compliance and the clinician–patient relationship: a review. *Social Science and Medicine.* **15**: 215–22.

Gibbons JS, Horn SH, Powell JM *et al.* (1984) Schizophrenic patients and their families: a survey in a psychiatric service based on a DGH Unit. *British Journal of Psychiatry.* **144**: 70–7.

Goffman E (1961) *Asylums.* Penguin, Harmondsworth.

Goldman HH (1982) Mental illness and family burden: a public health perspective. *Hospital and Community Psychiatry.* **33**: 557–60.

Gotzsche PC (1989) Methodology and overt and hidden bias in reports of 196 double-blind trials of nonsteroidal anti-inflammatory drugs in rheumatoid arthritis. *Controlled Clinical Trials.* **10**: 31–56.

Gournay K and Brooking J (1993) Failure and dissatisfaction. In: C Brooker and F White (eds) *Community Psychiatric Nursing: a research perspective. Volume 2.* Chapman and Hall, London.

Green M (1987) Women in the oppressor role: white racism. In: S Ernst and M Maguire (eds) *Living With The Sphinx: papers from the Women's Therapy Centre.* The Women's Press, London.

Greenberg JS, Greenley JR and Benedict P (1994) Contributions of persons with serious mental illness to their families. *Hospital and Community Psychiatry.* **45**: 475–80.

Greenwood E (1957) The attributes of a profession. *Social Work.* **2**(3): 45–55.

Grove B (1997) Mental health and employment: a personal view. *The Mental Health Review.* **2**: 5–7.

Guildford JP (1954) *Psychometric Methods.* McGraw-Hill, New York.

Hagan T and Smail D (1997) Power mapping: 1 Background and basic methodology. *Journal of Community and Applied Social Psychology.* **7**: 257–67.

Harp H (1991) *A Crazy Folks Guide to Reasonable Accommodations and Psychiatric Disability.* Center for Community Change through Housing and Support, Burlington, VT.

Hartmann PE and Becker MH (1978) Noncompliance with prescribed regimen among chronic hemodialysis patients: a method of prediction and educational diagnosis. *Dialysis and Transplantation.* **7**: 978–89.

Hatfield AB, Spaniol L and Zipple AM (1987) Expressed emotion: a family perspective. *Schizophrenia Bulletin.* **13**: 221–6.

Haynes RB, Taylor DW and Sackett DL (eds) (1979) *Compliance in Health Care.* Johns Hopkins University Press, Baltimore, MD.

Heinzelman F (1962) Determinants of prophylaxis behavior with respect to rheumatic fever. *Journal of Health and Human Behaviour.* **3**: 73–81.

Hirsch S, Craig T, Dean C *et al.* (1992) *Facilities and Services for the Mentally Ill with Persisting Severe Disabilities.* Working Party Report for the Royal College of Psychiatrists.

Hirsch SR and Leff JP (1975) *Abnormalities in Parents of Schizophrenics.* Maudsley Monograph No 22. Oxford University Press, London.

Hogarty GE, Anderson CM and Reiss DJ (1986) Family psychoeducation, social skills training and maintenance chemotherapy in the aftercare treatment of schizophrenia I: one year effects of a controlled study on relapse and adjustment. *Archives of General Psychiatry.* **43**: 633–42.

Hogarty GE, Anderson CM, Reiss DJ *et al.* (1991) Family psychoeducation, social skills training and maintenance chemotherapy in the aftercare of schizophrenia II: two year effects of a controlled study on relapse and adjustment. *Archives of General Psychiatry.* **48**: 340–7.

Hogarty GE, Schooler NR, Ulrich R *et al.* (1979) Fluphenazine and social therapy in the aftercare of schizophrenic patients. *Archives of General Psychiatry.* **36**: 1283–94.

Hoge SK, Applebaum PS, Lawlor T *et al.* (1990) A prospective, multi-centre study of patients' refusal of antipsychotic medication. *Archives of General Psychiatry.* **47**: 949–56.

Holden DF and Levine RRJ (1982) How families evaluate mental health professionals, resources and effects of illness. *Schizophrenia Bulletin.* **8**: 626–33.

Honig A, Pop P, Dekemp E *et al.* (1992) Physical illness in chronic psychiatric patients from a community unit revisited: a three year follow up study. *British Journal of Psychiatry.* **161**: 80–3.

Hoult J (1986) Community care of the acutely mentally ill. *British Journal of Psychiatry.* **149**: 137–44.

Jamison KR (1995) *An Unquiet Mind.* Alfred A Knopf, New York.

Janz NK and Becker MH (1984) The health belief model: a decade later. *Health Education Quarterly.* **11**: 1–47.

Johannsen WJ (1969) Attitudes towards mental patients: review of empirical research. *Mental Hygiene.* **53**(2): 218–28.

Jones K (1972) *A History of Mental Health Services.* Routledge and Keegan Paul, London.

Karasu TB (1986) The specificity vs non-specificity dilemmas: towards identifying therapeutic change agents. *American Journal of Psychiatry.* **143**: 687–95.

Kasl SV and Cobb S (1966) Health behaviour, illness behaviour and sick role behaviour. *Archives of Environmental Health.* **12**: 246–66 and 531–41.

Kazdin AE (1982) *Single-case research designs: methods for clinical and applied settings.* Oxford University Press, New York.

Kemp R, Hayward P, Applewhaite G *et al.* (1996) Compliance therapy in psychotic patients: randomised controlled trial. *British Medical Journal.* **312**: 315–19.

Kent S and Yellowlees P (1994) Psychiatric and social reasons for frequent rehospitalisation. *Hospital and Community Psychiatry.* **45**(4): 347–50.

Kirscht JP and Rosenstock IM (1977) Patient adherence to antihypertensive medical regimens. *Journal of Community Health.* **3**: 115–24.

Kitzinger J (1995) Introducing focus groups. *British Medical Journal.* **311**: 299–302.

Kitzinger C and Perkins R (1993) *Changing our Minds: lesbian feminism and psychology.* Only-women Press Ltd, London.

Kramarae C and Teichler PA (1985) *A Feminist Dictionary.* Pandora Press, London.

Kuipers L and Bebbington PE (1990) *Working in Partnership: clinicians and carers in the management of long-standing mental illness.* Heinemann, Oxford.

Laing RD and Esterson A (1964) *Sanity, Madness and the Family.* Penguin, Harmondsworth.

Lake RW (1983) Planners' alchemy: transforming NIMBY to YIMBY. *Journal of the American Planning Association.* **59**(1): 87–93.

Leader A (1995) *Direct Power.* Pavilion Publishing, Brighton.

Leete E (1988) *The Role of the Consumer Movement and People with Mental Illness.* Presentation at the *12th Mary Switzer Memorial Seminar in Rehabilitation.* Washington DC, June 15–16.

Leff J and Vaughn CE (1985) *Expressed Emotion in Families.* Guildford Press, New York.

Leff J, Kuipers L, Berkowitz R *et al.* (1982) A controlled trial of social intervention in the families of schizophrenic patients. *British Journal of Psychiatry.* **141**: 121–34.

Leff JP, Kuipers L, Berkowitz R *et al.* (1985) A controlled trial of social intervention on schizophrenia families: two years follow-up. *British Journal of Psychiatry.* **146**: 594–600.

Lefley HP (1989) Family burden and family stigma in major mental illness. *American Psychologist.* **44**: 556–60.

Lehman AF (1995) Vocational rehabilitation in schizophrenia. *Schizophrenia Bulletin.* **21**: 645–56.

Leventhal H, Diefenbach M and Leventhal EA (1992) Illness cognitions: using common sense to understand treatment adherence and affect-cognition interactions. *Cognitive Therapy and Research.* **16**: 143–63.

Lewis A (1934) The psychopathology of insight. *British Journal of Medical Psychology.* **14**: 332–48.

Lidz RW and Lidz T (1949) The family environment of schizophrenic patients. *American Journal of Psychiatry*. **106**: 332–45.

Lindow V (1994) *Purchasing Mental Health Services: self-help alternatives*. MIND Publications, London.

Lindow V (1996) What we want from community psychiatric nurses. In: J Read and J Reynolds (eds) *Speaking Our Minds*. Open University Press, Milton Keynes.

Luborsky L, Auerbach AH, Chandler M *et al.* (1971) Factors influencing the outcome of psychotherapy. *Psychological Bulletin*. **75**: 145–85.

Luborsky L, Crits-Cristoph P, Alexander L *et al.* (1983) Two helping alliance methods for predicting outcomes of psychotherapy. A counting signs vs. global rating method. *Journal of Nervous and Mental Disease*. **171**: 480–9.

Lucksted A and Coursey RD (1995) Consumer perceptions of pressure and force in psychiatric treatments. *Psychiatric Services*. **46**: 146–52.

Lynch MM and Kruzich JM (1986) Needs assessment of the chronically mentally ill: practitioner and client perspectives. *Administration in Mental Health*. **4**: 237–42.

McGuire A, Henderson J and Mooney G (1988) *The Economics of Health Care: an introductory text*. Routledge, London.

Macmillan JF, Crow TJ, Johnson AL *et al.* (1986) The Northwick Park first episodes of schizophrenia study. *British Journal of Psychiatry*. **148**: 128–33.

MacPherson R, Jerrom B and Hughes A (1997) Drug refusal among schizophrenic patients treated in the community. *Journal of Mental Health*. **6**: 141–7.

Manic Depression Fellowship (1995) *Inside Out: a guide to the self management of manic depression*. Manic Depression Fellowship, Kingston upon Thames.

Mann JJ (1986) How medication compliance affects outcome. *Psychiatric Annals*. **16**: 567–70.

Marsh DT (1992) *Families and Mental Illness: new directions in professional practice*. Praeger, New York.

Maslow A (1970) *The Assessment of Need*. Viking, London.

Masson J (1988) *Against Therapy*. Fontana/Collins, London.

Mechanic D (1972) Social psychologic factors affecting the presentation of bodily complaints. *New England Journal of Medicine*. **286**: 1132–9.

Meddings S (1997) *Service users' perspectives on the roles of different professionals in rehabilitation and continuing care*. Research submitted in part fulfilment of the requirements for the degree of Doctor of Clinical Psychology, University of Leicester.

Meltzer D, Hale AS, Malik SJ *et al.* (1991) Community care for patients with schizophrenia one year after discharge. *British Medical Journal*. **303**: 1023–6.

Meltzof J and Kornreich M (1970) *Research in Psychotherapy*. Atherton, New York.

Mendel WM (1986) Psychiatric treatment outcome research. *International Journal of Partial Hospitalisation*. **3**: 151–7.

Miller WR (1994) Motivational interviewing III. On the ethics of motivational intervention. *Behavioural and Cognitive Psychotherapy*. **22**: 111–23.

Miller WR (1995) The ethics of motivational interviewing revisited. *Behavioural and Cognitive Psychotherapy*. **23**: 345–8.

Miller FE (1996) Grief therapy for relatives of persons with serious mental illness. *Psychiatric Services*. **47**(6): 633–7.

MIND (1986) *Policy Paper on Women and Mental Health.* MIND Publications, London.

MIND (1993) *Submission of MIND (National Association for Mental Health) to the Mental Health Committee Inquiry into implications of any extension of legal powers under the Mental Health Act 1983 for the care of people with a mental illness in the community.* MIND Publications, London.

Mirin SM and Namerow SM (1991) Why study treatment outcome? *Hospital and Community Psychiatry*. **42**: 1007–13.

Mitchell JE, Pyle RL and Hatsukami D (1983) A comparative analysis of psychiatric problems listed by patients and physicians. *Hospital and Community Psychiatry*. **34**: 848–9.

Moodley P and Perkins R (1991) Routes to care in an inner city London borough. *Social Psychiatry and Social Epidemiology*. **26**: 47–51.

Mueser KT, Glynn SM, Corrigan PW *et al.* (1996) A survey of preferred terms for users of mental health services. *Psychiatric Services.* **47**: 760–1.

Muijen M and Hadley T (1995) The incentives war. *Health Service Journal*. **9 March**: 24–6.

Nibert D, Cooper S and Crossmaker M (1989) Assaults against residents of psychiatric institutions. *Journal of Interpersonal Violence*. **4**: 342-9.

O'Hagan M (1991) *Stopovers on My Way Home from Mars*. Survivors Speak Out, London.

O'Hagan M (1996) Two accounts of mental distress. In: J Read and J Reynolds (eds) *Speaking Our Minds*. Open University Press, Milton Keynes.

Onyett S, Pillinger T and Muijen M (1995) *Making Community Mental Health Teams Work: CMHTs and the people who work in them.* Sainsbury Centre for Mental Health, London.

Orbach S (1982) *Fat is a Feminist Issue.* Hamlyn, London.

Orbach S (1996) Couching anxieties. In: S Dunant and R Porter (eds) *The Age of Anxiety*. Virago Press, London.

Owen S (1997) Personal communication.

Panorama (1997) *A risk worth taking?* BBC1, 13 October.

Pembroke L (1997) *Who Is Harming Who?* National Self-Harm Network, London.

Perkins R (1993) *Twelve States and Twenty-Two Beds: a tour of innovative North American community care services for people with serious ongoing mental health problems*. Winston Churchill Travelling Fellowship Report, London.

Perkins R (1994) Choosing ECT. *Feminism and Psychology*. **4**: 623–6.

Perkins RE (1996a) Working with users. In: K Thompson and G Strathdee (eds) *Effectively Managing Mental Health Service Development*. Sainsbury Centre for Mental Health, London.

Perkins R (1996b) Seen but not heard: can 'user involvement' become more than empty rhetoric. *The Mental Health Review*. **1**: 16–19.

Perkins RE (1997) *Rehabilitation and Continuing Care Service: annual report and multidisciplinary audit*. Pathfinder Mental Health Services NHS Trust, London.

Perkins R and Dilks S (1992) Worlds apart: working with severely socially disabled people. *Journal of Mental Health*. **1**: 3–17.

Perkins R and Fisher NR (1996) Beyond mere existence: the auditing of care plans. *Journal of Mental Health*. **5**(3): 275–86.

Perkins R and Moodley P (1993) The arrogance of insight? *Psychiatric Bulletin*. **17**: 233–4.

Perkins RE and Repper JM (1996) *Working Alongside People With Serious Long-term Mental Health Problems*. Chapman and Hall, London.

Perkins R and Twelftree H (1997) *Long Term Care Case Register Report 1997*. Pathfinder Mental Health Services NHS Trust, London.

Perkins R, Buckfield R and Choy D (1997) Access to employment: a supported employment project to enable mental health service users to obtain jobs within mental health services. *Journal of Mental Health*. **6**(3): 307–18.

Perkins R, Nadirshaw Z, Copperman J *et al.* (eds) *Women in Context: good practice in mental health services for women*. GPMH, London.

Petrila JP and Sadoff RL (1992) Confidentiality and the family as caregiver. *Hospital and Community Psychiatry*. **43**: 136–9.

Phelan M, Slade M and Thornicroft G (1995) The Camberwell Assessment of Need. *British Journal of Psychiatry*. **167**: 598.

Philo G, Henderson L and McLaughlin G (1994a) *Mass media representations of mental health/illness*. Report to the Scottish Health Education Board. The Glasgow University Media Group, Glasgow.

Philo G, Henderson L and McLaughlin G (1994b) *Mass media representations of mental health/illness: audience responses*. Report to the Scottish Health Education Board. The Glasgow University Media Group, Glasgow.

Platt S and Kreitman N (1984) Trends in parasuicide and unemployment among men in Edinburgh, 1968-1982. *British Medical Journal*. **289**: 1029–32.

Pratt P (1998) The administration and monitoring of neuroleptic medication. In: C Brooker and J Repper (eds) *Policy, Practice and Research in Community Mental Health Services*. Bailliere Tindall, London.

Podell RN (1975) *Physician's Guide to Compliance in Hypertension*. Merck, Rahway, NJ.

Powell R and Slade M (1995) Defining severe mental illness. In: G Thornicroft and G Strathdee (eds) *Purchasing Mental Health Services*. Cambridge University Press, London.

Rapp C and Wintersteen R (1989) The strengths model: results from 12 demonstrations. *Psycho-social Rehabilitation*. **13**: 23–32.

Read J (1996) What do we want from mental health services? In: J Read and J Reynolds (eds) *Speaking Our Minds*. Open University Press. Milton Keynes.

Read J (1997) What is a good day project? *A Life in the Day*. **1**: 7–11.

Read J and Reynolds J (eds) (1996) *Speaking Our Minds*. Open University Press, Milton Keynes.

Reed C (1990) I am a Californian, therefore I dream. *Guardian*. **April 13**: 8.

Repper J and Brooker C (1996) Attitudes towards community facilities for people with serious mental health problems. *Health and Social Care in the Community*. 4(5): 290–399.

Repper J and Brooker C (1998) Difficulties in the measurement of outcome in people who have serious mental health problems. *Journal of Advanced Nursing*. In press.

Repper J and Perkins R (1994) Targeting a local service for the severely mentally ill: implications for CPNs. In: C Brooker and E White (eds) *Community Psychiatric Nursing: a research perspective. Volume 3*. Chapman and Hall, London.

Repper J and Perkins R (1995) Meeting the needs of neglected patients. *Nursing Standard*. **9**: 28–31.

Repper J, Perkins R and Owen S (1998) 'I wanted to be a nurse ... but I didn't get that far'. Women with serious ongoing mental health problems speak about their lives. Submitted to *Journal of Psychiatric and Mental Health Nursing*.

Repper J, Sayce L, Strong S *et al.* (1997) *Tall Stories from the Backyard: a national survey of local NIMBY opposition to community mental health facilities*. Mind Publications, London.

Ridgeway P (1988) *The Voice of Consumers in Mental Health Systems: a call for change*. Centre for Community Change through Housing and Support, Burlington, VT.

Rogers ES and Palmer-Erbs V (1994) Participatory action research: implications for researchers in psychiatric rehabilitation. *Psychosocial Rehabilitation Journal*. **18**: 3–12.

Rogers A, Pilgrim D and Lacey R (1993) *Experiencing Psychiatry: users' views of services*. Macmillan, Basingstoke.

Rogers ES, Chamberlin J, Ellison ML *et al.* (1997) A consumer-constructed scale to measure empowerment among users of mental health services. *Psychiatric Services*. **48**: 1042–7.

Rollnick S and Miller WR (1995) What is motivational interviewing? *Behavioural and Cognitive Psychotherapy*. **23**: 325–34.

Rose D (1996) *Living in the Community*. Sainsbury Centre for Mental Health, London.

Rose N (1989) Individualizing psychology. In: J Shotter and KJ Gergen (eds) *Texts of Identity*. Sage Publications, London.

Rowland L and Perkins RE (1988) You can't eat, drink and make love eight hours a day: the value of work in psychiatry. *Health Trends.* **20**: 75–9.

Royal College of Psychiatrists (1987) *Community Treatment Orders: a discussion document*. Royal College of Psychiatrists, London.

Royal College of Psychiatrists and College of Occupational Therapists (1992) *A Consensus Statement: occupational therapy and mental disorders*. Royal College of Psychiatrists and College of Occupational Therapists, London.

Royal College of Psychiatrists (1993a) *Patient Factsheet: ECT*. Royal College of Psychiatrists, London.

Royal College of Psychiatrists (1993b) *The Royal College Calls for an Amendment to the Mental Health Act 1983: 'Community Supervision Order'* (Press Release). Royal College of Psychiatrists, London.

Royal College of Psychiatrists (1996) *Report of the Confidential Inquiry into Homicides and Suicides by Mentally Ill People*. Royal College of Psychiatrists, London.

Ruggeri M (1994) Patients' and relatives' satisfaction with psychiatric services: the state of the art of its measurement. *Social Psychiatry and Psychiatric Epidemiology.* **29**: 212–27.

Ruscher SM, de Wit R and Mazmanian D (1997) Psychiatric patients' attitudes about medication and factors affecting noncompliance. *Psychiatric Services.* **48**: 82–5.

Ryan P (1986) Noncompliance. In: JM Thompson, GK McFarland, JE Hirsch *et al.* (eds) *Clinical Nursing*. The CV Mosby Company, St Louis, MO.

Sackett DL (1976) The magnitude of compliance and non-compliance. In: DL Sackett and RB Haynes (eds) *Compliance with Therapeutic Regimens*. Johns Hopkins University Press, Baltimore, MD.

Sandford T (1996) Involving users in depot phenothiazine services. In: T Sandford and K Gournay (eds) *Perspectives in Mental Health Nursing*. Bailliere Tindall, London.

Sang B and O'Brien J (1984) *Advocacy: the UK and American experience*. King's Fund, London.

Sainsbury Centre for Mental Health (1997) *Pulling Together: the future roles and training of mental health staff*. Sainsbury Centre for Mental Health, London.

Sayce LL (1998) *From Psychiatric Patient to Citizen*. MacMillan, London.

Scheff TJ (1966) *Being Mentally Ill: a sociological theory*. Aldine, Chicago.

Scheff TJ (1975) *Labelling Madness*. Prentice-Hall, Englewood Cliffs, NJ.

Scheme AH, Tessler RC and Gamache GM (1994) Instruments for measuring family or caregiver burden in severe mental illness. *Social Psychiatry and Psychiatric Epidemiology.* **28**: 11–16.

Seltzer A, Roncari I and Garfinkel P (1980) Effect of patient education on medication compliance. *American Journal of Psychiatry.* **25**: 638–45.

Shepherd G (1984) *Institutional Care and Rehabilitation.* Longman Applied Psychology, London.

Shepherd G (1990) Case management. *Health Trends.* **22**: 59–61.

Shepherd G, Murray A and Muijen M (1994) *Relative Values: the differing views of users, family carers and professionals on services for people with schizophrenia in the community.* The Sainsbury Centre for Mental Health, London.

Shepherd G, Murray A and Muijen M (1995) Perspectives on schizophrenia: a survey of user, family care and professional views regarding effective care. *Journal of Mental Health.* **4**: 403–22.

Sherlock R (1986) My brother's keeper? Mental health policy and the new psychiatry. In: DK Kentsmith, S Salladay and Mya PA (eds) *Ethics in Mental Health Practice.* Grune and Stratton, New York.

Smith R (1985) 'I'm just not right': the physical health of the unemployed. *British Medical Journal.* **291**: 1626–9.

Srebnick D, Robinson M and Tanzman BH (1990) *Participation of Mental Health Consumers in Research: empowerment in practice.* Poster Session, American Psychological Association Convention, Boston, MA.

Steele K (1992) Patients as experts: consumer appraisal of health services. *Public Money and Mamagement.* **October–December** issue.

Stein LI and Test MA (1980) Alternatives to mental hospital 1: treatment programme and clinical evaluation. *Archives of General Psychiatry.* **37**: 117–79.

Steinem G (1992) *Revolution from Within: a book of self-esteem.* Bloomsbury, London.

Strauss JS (1994) The person with schizophrenia as a person II: approaches to the subjective and complex. *British Journal of Psychiatry.* **164** (suppl 23): 103–7.

Szmukler G (1996) From family 'burden' to caregiving. *Psychiatric Bulletin.* **20**: 449–51.

Tanzman B (1993) An overview of surveys of mental health consumers' preferences for housing and support services. *Hospital and Community Psychiatry.* **44**: 5.

Taylor B (1996) Reflections on therapy. In: J Read and J Reynolds (eds) *Speaking Our Minds.* Open University Press, Milton Keynes.

Taylor KE and Perkins RE (1991) Identity and coping with mental illness in long-stay psychiatric rehabilitation. *British Journal of Clinical Psychology.* **30**: 50–1.

Taylor L (1996) ECT is barbaric. In: J Read and J Reynolds (eds) *Speaking Our Minds.* Open University Press, Milton Keynes.

Thompson C (1996) *Letter to the Committee from the Royal College of Psychiatrists (ICB 20).* House of Commons Social Security Committee. Session 1996–97.

Thompson EH (1988) Variation in the self-concept of young adult chronic patients: chronicity reconsidered. *Hospital and Community Psychiatry.* **39**: 260–4.

Thompson EH and Doll W (1982) The burden of families coping with the mentally ill: an invisible crisis. *Family Relations*. **31**: 379–88.

Thompson R (1993a) Letter to Deborah Reidy, Director, Education for Community Initiatives. Bethesda, MD.

Thompson R (1993b) *News analysis: July 10th*. Bethesda, MD.

Thompson R (1993c) Activities that George Orwell would have understood perfectly. *News analysis: January 28th*. Bethesda, MD.

Thompson R (1993d) Letter to Frederick Goodwin, Director, National Institute of Mental Health. Betheseda, MD.

Titelman D (1991) Grief, guilt and identification in siblings of schizophrenic individuals. *Bulletin of the Menninger Clinic*. **55**: 72–84.

Torrey EF (1986) Finally, a cure for the homeless: but it takes some strong medicine. *The Washington Monthly*. **10**: 95–7.

Tossell D and Webb R (1994) *Inside the Caring Services* (2nd edition). Edward Arnold, London.

Tyrer P, Smith J and Adshead G (1994) Ethical dilemmas in drug treatments. *Psychiatric Bulletin*. **18**: 203–4.

Tyrer P, Higgs R and Strathdee G (1993) *Mental Health and Primary Care: a changing agenda*. Gaskell and the Mental Health Foundation, London.

Vaughn CE and Leff JP (1976) The influence of family and social factors on the course of mental illness. *British Journal of Psychiatry*. **129**: 125–37.

Vaughn CE and Leff JP (1981) Patterns of emotional response in relatives of schizophrenic patients. *Schizophrenia Bulletin*. **7**: 43–5.

Walker M (1989) It's floating death out there and they want to talk dollars. *Guardian*. **April 15**: 23.

Walshe K and Ham C (1997) *Acting on the Evidence: progress in the NHS*. University of Birmingham Health Services Management Centre/The NHS Confederation, Birmingham.

Warner R (1985) *Recovery from Schizophrenia: psychiatry and political economy*. Routledge and Keegan Paul, London.

Warner R, Taylor D, Powers M *et al.* (1989) Acceptance of the mental illness label by psychotic patients: effects on functioning. *American Journal of Orthopsychiatry*. **59**(3): 398–409.

Watts F and Bennett D (eds) (1983) *Theory and Practice of Psychiatric Rehabilitation*. Wiley, Chichester.

Williams A (1978) Need as an economic exegesis. In: AJ Culyer and KG Wright (eds) *Economic Aspects of Health Services*. Martin Robertson, Oxford.

Williams J and Watson G (1994) Mental health services that empower women: the challenge to clinical psychology. *Clinical Psychology Forum*. **64**: 6–12.

Willis MJ (1982) The impact of schizophrenia on families: one mother's point of view. *Schizophrenia Bulletin.* **8**: 617–19.

Winefield H and Burnett P (1996) Barriers to an alliance between family and professional caregivers in chronic schizophrenia. *Journal of Mental Health.* **5**: 223–32.

Wing JK (1978) Clinical concepts of schizophrenia. In: JK Wing (ed) *Schizophrenia: towards a new synthesis.* Academic Press, London.

Wing JK (1962) Institutionalism in mental hospitals. *British Journal of Social and Clinical Psychology.* **1**: 38–51.

Wing JK and Brown GW (1970) *Institutionalism and Schizophrenia.* Cambridge University Press, London.

Wing JK and Morris B (1981) *Handbook of Psychiatric Rehabilitation.* Oxford University Press, Oxford.

Withers JMJ (1995) Motivational interviewing: a special ethical dilemma? *Behavioural and Cognitive Psychotherapy.* **23**: 335–9.

Wood D and Copperman J (1996) Sexual harassment and assault in psychiatric settings. In: R Perkins, Z Nadirshaw, J Copperman *et al.* (eds) *Women in Context: good practice in mental health services for women.* GPMH, London.

World Health Organisation (1965) *Aspects of Family Mental Health in Europe.* World Health Organisation, Geneva.

Wynne LC and Singer MT (1963) Thought disorder and family relationships of schizophrenics II: a classification of forms of thinking. *Archives of General Psychiatry.* **9**: 199–206.

Wolfensburger W and Tullman S (1982) A brief outline of the principle of normalisation. *Rehabilitation Psychology.* **27**: 131–45.

Zito Trust (1995) *Learning the Lessons.* Zito Trust, London.

Index